I0114539

Knightly Weaponry Play
The Manual of Fencing and Archery for German Scouting

The Manual of Fencing and Archery for German Scouting

Knightly Weaponry Play

Written and Illustrated by

WILHELM FABRICIUS

Translated and Edited by

JEFFREY HULL

ANTELOPE HILL PUBLISHING

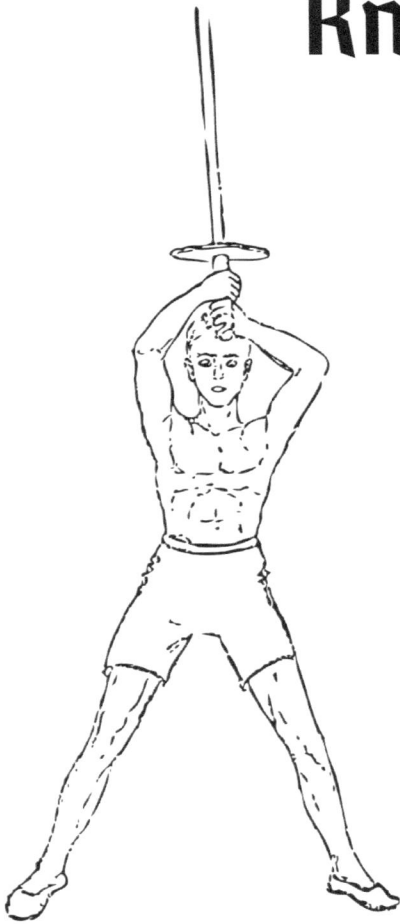

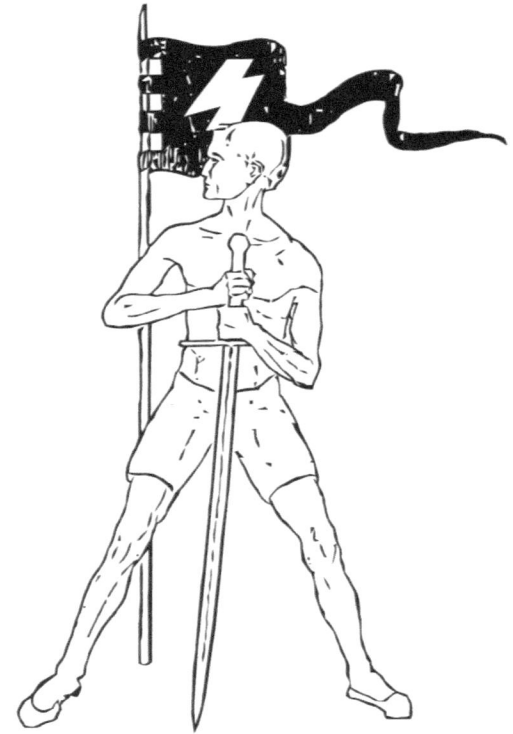

Copyright © 2021 Jeffrey Hull

Second printing 2021.

Originally *Ritterliche Waffenspiele, Schwert- und Stockfechten, Bogenschießen, Armbrustschießen, Bau von Übungswaffen etc.* by Wilhelm Fabricius, published by Holzinger: Stuttgart 1935 (2nd edition).

Translated 2017 by Jeffrey Hull.
This edition published by Antelope Hill Publishing, 2021.

Cover art by sswifty.
Interior formatting by Margaret Bauer.

The publisher can be contacted at:
Antelopehillpublishing.com

Hardcover ISBN-13: 978-1-953730-95-4

Disclaimer: The use of the techniques described in this book, even with soft weapons designed for safety, is an inherently dangerous activity. It can result in serious injury, especially for inexperienced users. When practicing these techniques, the use of protective equipment and reasonable caution is strongly advised, and sparring should always be done in a supervised setting. The publishers, translators, or authors of this work are not responsible for any injuries proceeding from the use of any of the techniques described herein.

I dedicate this work to my wonderful son

-JH

Contents

Translator's Foreword

This is an instructional manual for the basic, fun, and clever wielding by youth of longsword, single stick, bow and arrow, and crossbow and bolt. Published in Germany in 1935 as Ritterliche Waffenspiele (Knightly Weaponry Play), this second edition book was originally written by a patriotic forester, naturalist, and Scouting leader, Herr-Doktor Wilhelm Fabricius, who along with his faithful wife, Frau Anna Schweickhardt, worked to inspire their nation's various juvenile environmental-survival fellowships and brotherhoods like Deutsche Freischar, Wandervögel, Deutsche Jungenschaft, Adler und Falken, Deutsches Jungvolk, Bündische Jugend, Pfadfinder (German Volunteers, Wandering Birds, German Youngship, Eagle and Falcons, German Youngfolk, League of Youth, Path-Finders = Scouts). This little field manual, now exceedingly rare, was the combined 23rd/24th final volume of the once-popular series of the chocolate-bar-sized Scouting Rucksack-Bücherei (rucksack-library), codicologically remarkable for their finely wrought pictures and bold yet delicate fonts, plus archival quality paper and sturdy bindings.

Fabricius evidently wanted the German youth of his day to learn something of the noble and manly arts of combat pursued by Medieval German Ritter (knights). Indeed, his book's swordplay clearly interprets moves of Kunst des Fechtens (art of fencing/fighting) as illustrated centuries earlier by venerable Fechtmeister (fencing/fight-masters) like Hans Talhoffer (1467) and Joachim Meyer (1570 and 1600), and a probable Fechter and Ringer (fencer and wrestler) like Albrecht Dürer (1512). All such were constituents of the array of martial arts correctly known as Ritterlich Kunst (Knightly/Chivalric Arts). Howsoever imperfect his interpretation of those past teachings might be, Fabricius made up for it by his motivational vitality.

The goal of this book is juvenile martial prowess, which is the organic outcome of suprarational self-worth and historical curiosity leading to autodidactic achievement. Training at such positive athletic activities makes for a higher quality citizen. These were specifically intended, along with a kaleidoscopic variety of other worthwhile activities, to help the Scouts make themselves from boys into men for the benefit of, and to the credit of, their Volksgemeinschaft (ethnic community: i.e. Germany = nation, people, culture). That said, weaponry play—with some vigorous wrestling along the way—simply makes for great joy!

Despite its original edifying intentions, this book has often been reviled for being a National Socialist publication. Indeed, it was usurped by that prevailing contemporary regime for purposes of educating and toughening boys eventually subsumed to its authority and responsibility, as started at regime ascendency in 1933. That is evinced by (1) a two-part official introduction by Path-Finder Branch-Director Wilhelm Fabricius and by Hitler-Youth Baden Leader Friedhelm Kemper, including obligatory salutations to Herr-Führer Adolf Hitler; and (2) one picture of an Aryan youth standing before the triangular monochrome S-rune pennon of the Deutsches Jungvolk (German Youngfolk). Otherwise, said introduction suggests years of play-testing and worth-proving of the fencing and archery by Scouts, which culminated at a major summertime jamboree in the southwestern march of Franconia in 1935. (See the two jamboree images at the very end of this work.)

In any event, the most valuable and eternal politics here are the metapolitics, whereby traditional martial arts were offered as a natural, cultural way for the betterment both of bold, German youth and of their dearly-held country. Thus this book admirably and rightfully shows normal, healthy, self-valuing German youth making themselves mighty by learning how to fight. It witnesses the enthusiasm of self-empowerment and the spirit of male bonding fostered by the various folkish youth movements of Germany, Austria, and Switzerland during better times of yore, when Europa still owned her dignity and her sovereignty.

Indeed this book is a most relevant and dynamic bequeathal for introducing all modern European youth to their ethno-cultural birthright of chivalric martial arts: For this heritage is theirs and always deserves to be theirs, inasmuch as they likewise make themselves deserving. May it guide them towards weaponizing themselves and protecting their beautiful and beloved maidens, as nowadays is desperately so needed. May these aforesaid European youth—wherever they may be upon this Earth—make positive nationalistic regeneracy beyond the negative globalist degeneracy forced upon them by modern schools, governments, finance, entertainment, and mass media. May they always and forever keep their pride and their ferocity. May these youth find their true selves and enjoy fulfilling lives, free and wild amid forests and fields, fighting with their swords in the light of the Sun. Indeed, today's European youth must be liberated of hatred for the past, and consequently for their own being, both which they did not create. They must be encouraged to love the future, and consequently their own becoming, both which they are to create, hopefully to their greater glory. Thusly may the activities of this book lead our beautiful and beloved youth towards a superior tomorrow!

- JH

Introduction

This book is a fencing book, only insofar as it is a broadly restrictive regulation of the wild usage of pickets or hazel dowels, as is needed for the fencer and weapon to endure the play for a while. Moreover, the play shall be aesthetic, thus equally wild and supple, not just rough. You kids shall strike each other hard, not thrash each other weakly! Therefore, put your entire love for athletics into the duel/combat. Additionally, I want to give you kids some encouragement.

The bowshooting regulations, however, must indeed be executed very similarly to what stands written here, or else the weapon is indeed quickly shattered, although not so fast that injurious misfortune could not simply happen first.

For all Chivalric Arts, breeding and order are equally self-evident as for all other HY-activity. And this regulation like any other was scarcely fabricated at some office desk. We have managed these things for years and now as "experts" have presently written them down. And yet we all live, unwounded, and no bumps and no welts can spoil our combative joy.
Youth Domain Settlement 2/112

Hail Hitler!
Hartmut*

We want to raise a courageous and hard generation of National Socialist youth. Our comrade, Branch-Director Wilhelm Fabricius, through his fencing play, has guided our youth towards a way for skill, fearlessness, and tough composure in combat. His contribution, in the words and pictures here, are the groundwork for that.
Southwestern March Camp (Jamboree), 1935

Hail Hitler!
Friedhelm Kemper

(UCLA Library cataloguing marks)   *Hartmut (Hard-Courage) was the fanciful Path-Finder name-of-honor for Wilhelm Fabricius.

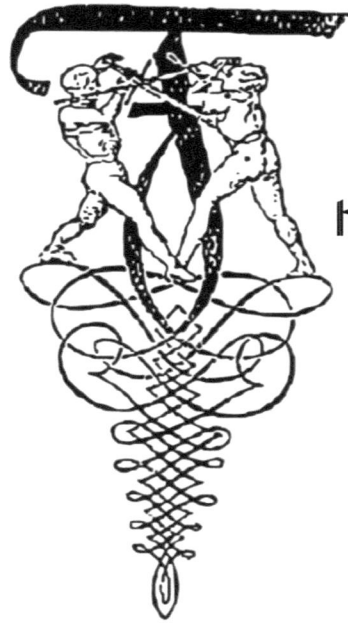

The Longsword: Fencing/Fighting

From old manuscripts, woodcuts, drawings, and engravings of "two-handed fencing" we have revealed unto ourselves what bespeaks our kind, and also what makes for unrestrained and dynamic joy: We, comrades of the great League of Youth.

It was stunt-work! Firstly, our fencing cannot be so artful as (Medieval/Renaissance guilds like) Saint Mark's Brothers and Free Fencers of the Feather practiced it during the 16th and 17th centuries, because indeed we do not exclusively dedicate ourselves thereto. Secondly, it ought not to be so uncouth as Landsknecht fencing, with its "good moves for each and every strong man," because we are not some power-sports union, and also the treachery of this fencing art would not then favor us. Thirdly, the fencing really ought to produce a few bruises, but no eye injuries and no bone fractures. (Which means that controlling one's own strikes is vital.) Thusly said, mothers always get it wrong to recognize us fencers without aid of identifying marks. Fourthly, it must be done (as pictured by old sources) without any protective gear, and with (affordable) self-made weapons.

The outcome is a mixture of fencing, dancing, and self-defensive wrestling. Our fencing requires speed and flexibility, self-control and momentum, some courage and temper, now daring then cunning. Either a guy totally partakes, body and mind, or else he gets constantly beaten!

The proper rules have varied according to goal and custom. We make our own selves. According to old archetypes, but concisely and with lots of room for personal art.

The principles designated as "Fight-Master Summary"* from Meyer fight-book, Straßburg circa 1600:

With these weapons reach wide and long,
After the hew afore thee overhang[1]
With thy body, and tread far thereto,[2]
Forcefully conduct thy hews around him here,[3]
To all four endings let those fly.
With gesturing and tugging thou him canst trick,[4]
At the blade-strong thou shalt intercept[5]
While with the blade-weak prevent him.
Indeed, nearer thou shalt not come,
Then that gets him with a hit.

When he would intrude you, then clear
The forward locus,[6] drive him from thee.
He warded thee but intruded:
Whoever with gripping and wrestling shall be first.
The strong and weak prevail evenly[7]—
Inthereof[8] makes the targets obvious;
Into before and after, correctly tread[9];
Keenly mark at the correct time;
And let thyself not be easily frightened!

*This is not exactly a "fight-master summary," because it was originally written as advice for fencing with the *dussack* (cutlass)—that said, however, this masterly advice is largely valid for the kinetics of longsword fencing. (Cf. Hull, 2012)

---

[1] Overhang with your body: you should reach as far as you can bow/lean forwards.

[2] Thereto tread far = lunge.

[3] "He/Him" is always the adversary (in context of fight-books—which in turn speak of "you/ye" as student(s) of the fight-master).

[4] Gesturing and tugging are explicit and implicit feints.

[5] The cuts of the adversary should become caught with the nearer (defensive) third of the sword. While with the further (offensive) two-thirds of the sword, you can often hit him at the same time.

[6] The Forward Locus is the forward half of your fencing zone—see figure of page 7 below.

[7] Perhaps called that, because you should negotiate the nature of adversary's fencing; for example, whether he fences strongly or weakly.

[8] "Inthereof" is the hew—during the adversary's too-slow attack—upon any of his open targets. For this "hew inthereof," special stepping and springing movements are needed. As well, corresponding steps for strike and counterstrike are to be made. (Hull, *Inthereof.*)

[9] That was clarified way back when with illustrations. (Hull, *Inthereof.*)

Fight-Summary for Us Today

You should fence with your adversary and to his body, and not with the adversary's sword and not to his weapon. You should not tap, rather hit, the adversary, with lots of swing, as if he actually stood in a wambeson. However, with the long hilt you can stop your hew just before hitting, so that he easily recovers despite your momentum.

The fencing entry and exit display guts and ingenuity; the engagement, the art, and the speed of the fencer; comprehension of the combative environment; and temper. Nimble, not timid, evasion is allowed, provided the adversary is kept in sight. All fencing is then only proper when it looks proud and good at every moment.

A wooden waster! Of the best ash wood.[11] Initially, when awkwardness leads to bruises and broken weapons, then accept pinewood. The entire weapon's length, including hilt, is 1.4 meters; breadth at the grip 4 cm; thickness 2 cm. The hilt should be 30 cm long and 3 cm thick, with a screwed-on wooden knob, the pommel. The oval cross is 17 cm long and at its middle 8 cm broad.

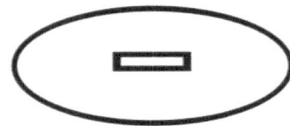

Overhead View

---

[10] Refer to Oakeshott, *Records of the Medieval Sword* and to Hull, *Early European Longswords* about that weapon.
[11] Best wood for spear-shafts too.

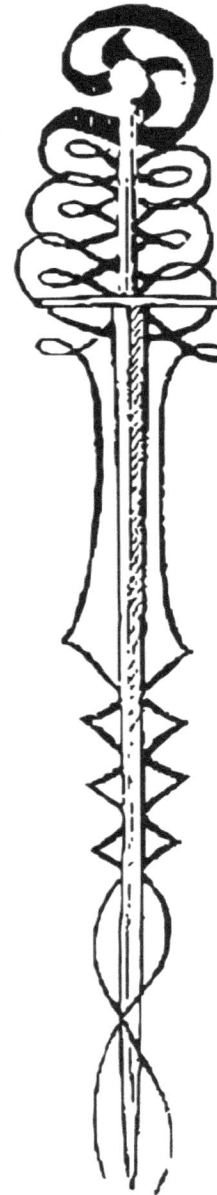

The Sword[10]

End-Knob = "Pommel"

Hand-Grip = "Hilt"

Hand-Guard = "Cross"

Near Third = "Strong"

Middle Third = "Half-Sword"

Far Third = "Weak"

Final Tip = "Point"

The Fencing Compass

All fencing has three parts: Entering, or the attack; Engaging, or the "winding" or the "hand-work"; and Exiting, or the withdrawal; which were all instructed by the past fight-masters (e.g. Meyer).

The fencing compass is drawn in the sand with the sword and whitened by the impartial fight-master. Firstly and uprightly, with both hands fastened at the pommel, he describes a circle around himself with the sword. That is the fencing zone for the one fencer. Then he treads onto that circumference and describes a second circle, which goes through the midpoint of the first. That is the fencing zone for the other fencer.

Each fencer treads from his side with one foot in his "locus." The middle, where the circles intersect, that is the "Forward Locus," wherein the engagement gets combatted. If a fencer succeeds at invading the Forward Locus of his adversary, who is not to be driven away by the sword, then he must be thrown out by combative wrestling. Thus exiting is the withdrawal up to the outer brink of one's own locus.

He has victory who drives the adversary out of his circle by "intruding" the Forward Locus; or who throws him out of the circles entirely by wrestling roundabout the Forward Locus.

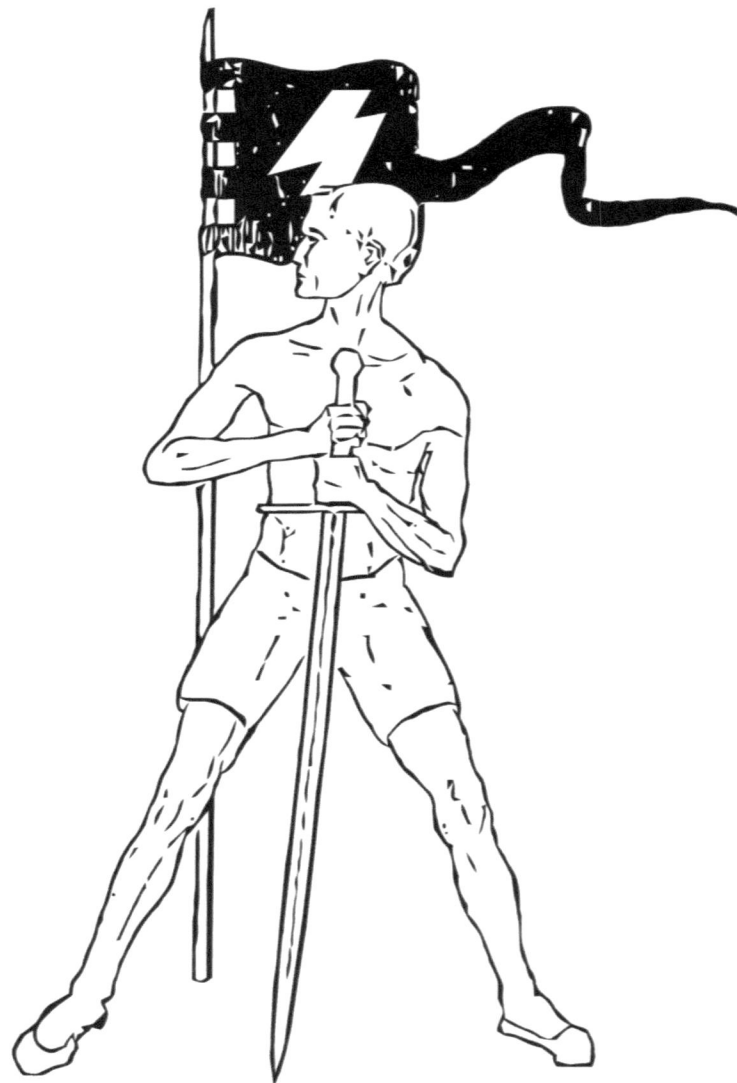

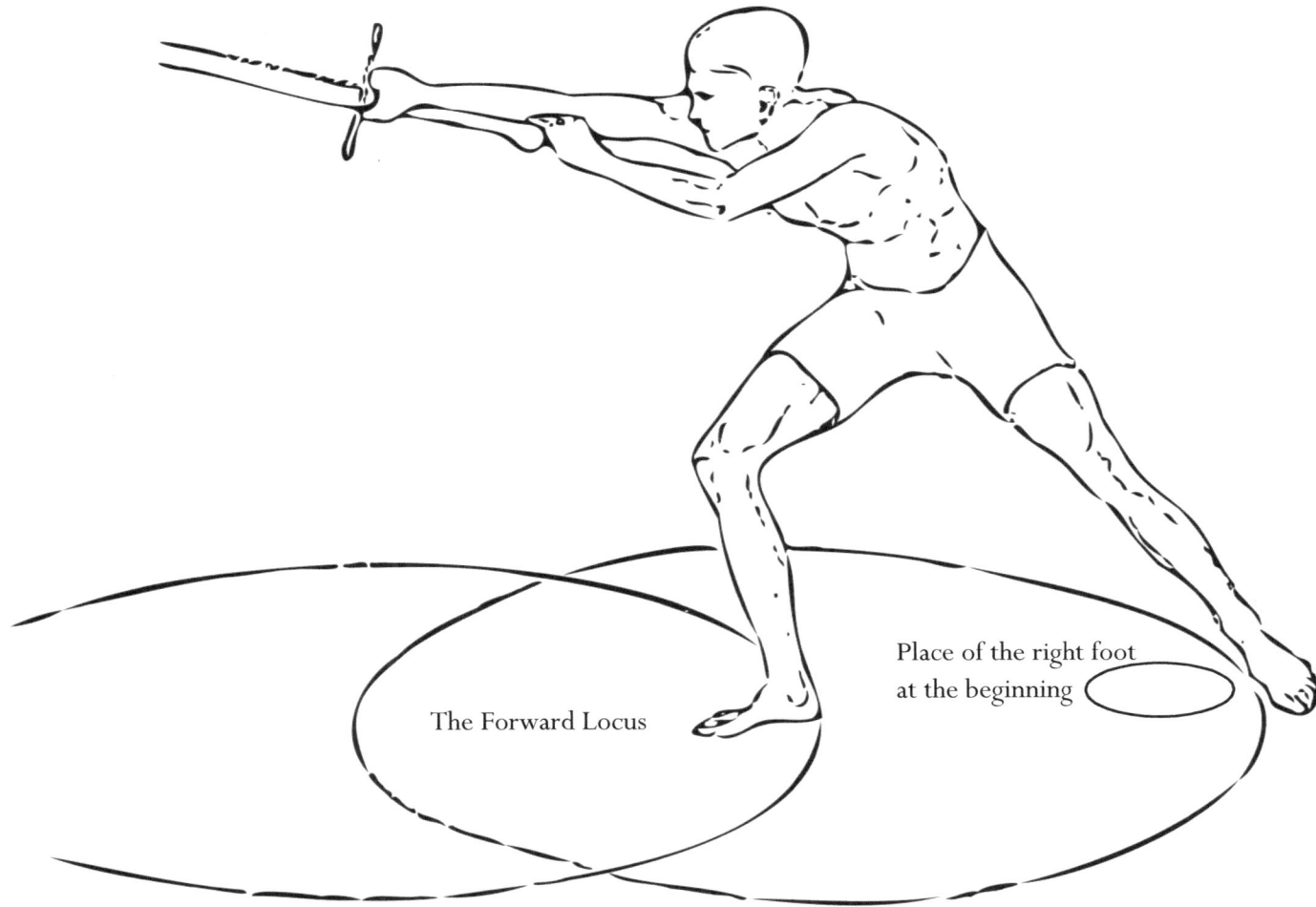

The Forward Locus

Place of the right foot
at the beginning

"Exchanging stances" during the fencing or wrestling, so that either combatant stands in the opposing circle, is allowed, even when it happens involuntarily. Naturally, the match can also be fought by hitscore.

Commencing, Saluting, Starting Stance

The fencer forms up one step before his circle, his sword shouldered at his right, his legs somewhat outspread, and his front towards his adversary.

For salute, he thrusts the weapon vertically high, and then swings one Wrath-Hew each towards right and left. The hews end again in the illustrated composure. The starting stance is an optional flourish, by which one foot treads into the "locus."

The Hews

The hews are swift circular swings. Those depend not upon weight, rather upon easy movements. The hits are strikes, not flicks. The only valid hits are those which speed across at least 1/4 of the circular arc, or which the adversary has consequently brought upon himself by flailing (e.g. Squint-Hew).

I.   All hews hewn from high to low are called "From the Day"[12] or Wrath-Hews.

1.   The "Skull-Hew" hits vertically from above upon the head or a shoulder or—by wide fencing distance—upon a forearm (e.g. Prime in sport-fencing).

---

[12] *Vom Tag* (From the Day) is the most basic longsword ward/stance traditionally taught by the Medieval German martial arts High Master Johann Liechtenauer.

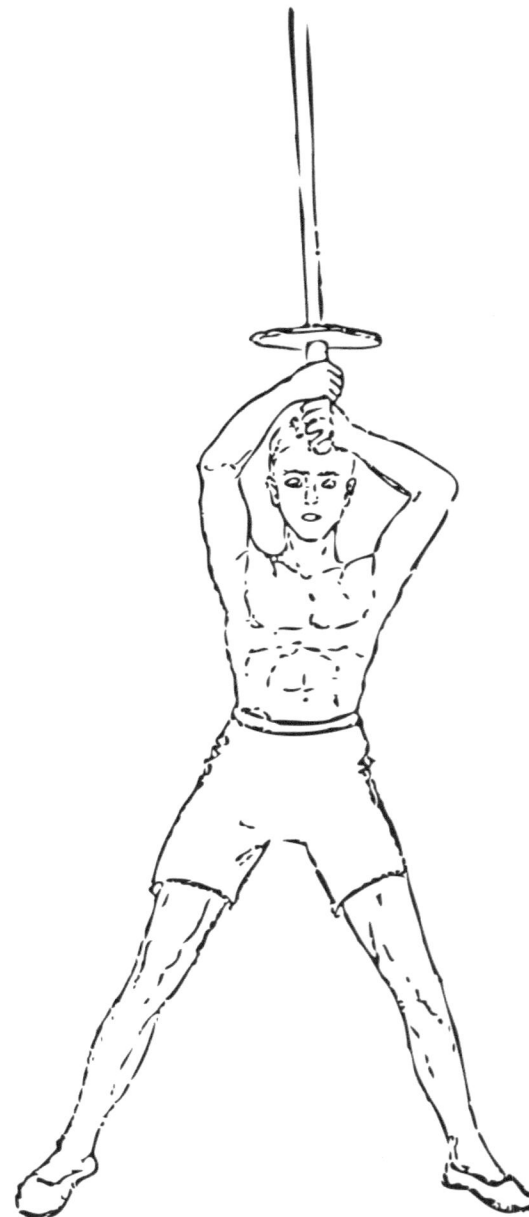

Skull Hew

Overhew Left

Overhew Right

Middlehew Left

Middlehew Right

Underhew Left

Underhew Right

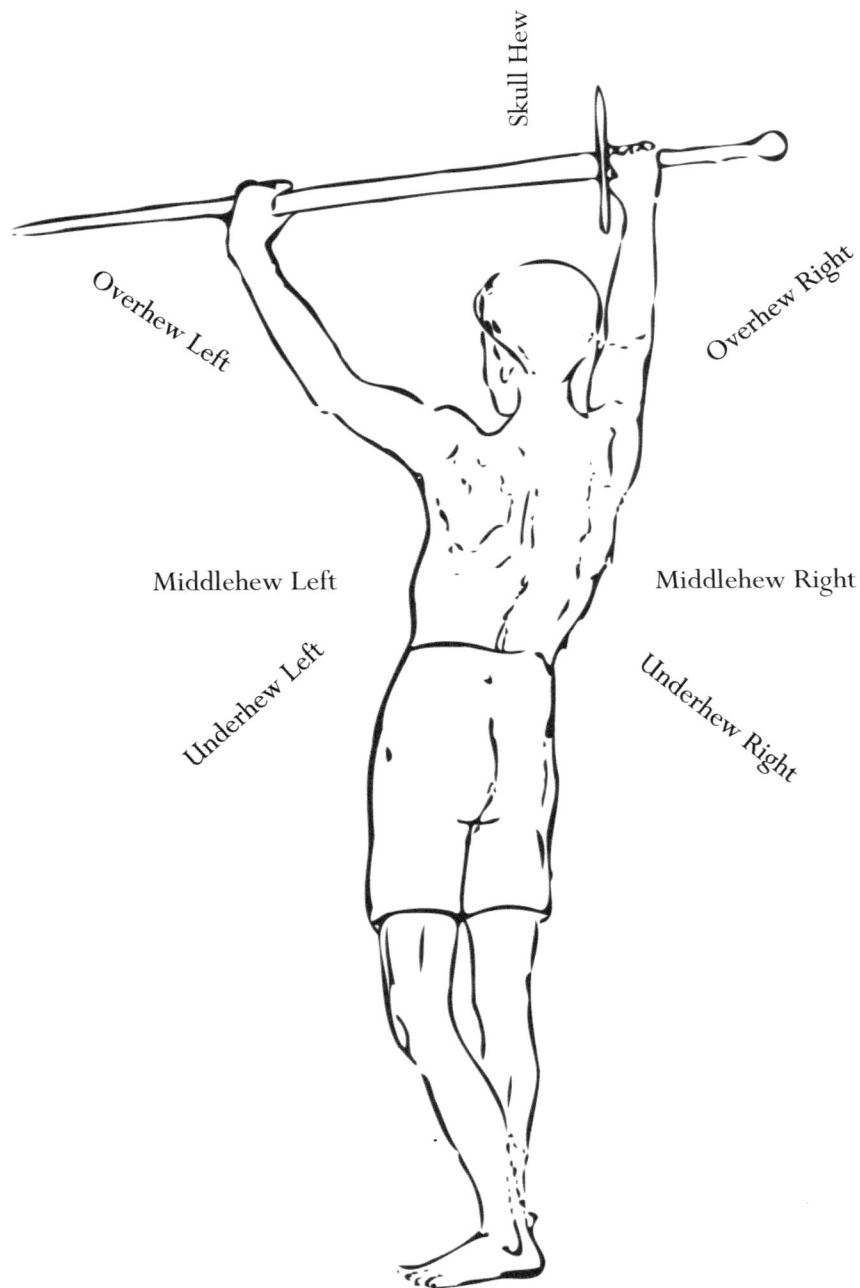

2. "Overhew Left" is a "twisted hew" with crossed arms which strikes diagonally from above, as Tierce hits.

3. "Overhew Right" is the Quarte striking diagonally from above upon ear, shoulder, or arm.[13]

II. The "Middlehews" are roughly horizontally-directed swings, equally Quarte and Tierce. They hit accordingly high from either side.

III. The "Underhews" are stricken diagonally from below, and hit either the flanks or the arms of the adversary from below.

There are not to be stabs or thrusts. Those are forbidden by us, even though it says in an old regulation: "And when he staggers, stab the sword into him." Likewise unlawful are strikes and thrusts with the hilting, cross, and pommel.

[13] Evidently, Fabricius' intended descriptions and comments for Overhews were misplaced in the layout of his book. I have corrected those mistakes by transposing them correctly within my translation. Now the names, descriptions, comments, and moves properly match.

Regarding special artful cuts—then read further beyond here—but only when you kids dominate the basic cuts.

The hit-areas are the entire body.

Yet it is profoundly unprofessional, and a signal of crudity and anxiety, to execute sniping-strikes to the adversary's hands or cheap-shots to his ankles.

Likewise, hews are to be shunned which shall only strike the weapon from the adversary's hands.

Those cost too much wood.

It commonly evinces good and secure fencing, when you allow the adversary the opportunity to execute a clean attack, which you can just as cleanly intercept, so then to swat the adversary within your counterstrike. Versus a slow or hesitant adversary, you may simply hew into his attack. But a hit by you only gets counted good if firstly it was a well-accelerated cut and not anxious fumbling, and if secondly you did not get hit thereby.

A "Fail-Hew" is a hew which shall not hit, rather misleading the adversary to make an unforeseen mismovement, whereby he exposes his targets. "Fail-Hew" means the Feint.

A "Squint-Hew" is an interception—a diversion—whereby the adversary himself hews your sword into his body. The adversary gets "invited" to the attack, when sideways you remove his sword with yours, and thereby expose your chest uncovered.

Interceptions

"Interception" means diverting with the Sword. To every hew belongs one corresponding interception.

How the interceptions are performed, emerges most clearly from the following illustrations.

The First Interception against all Wrath-Hews is done with the sword held straight overhead. This is the safest, yet also the slowest for ongoing fencing, and is the "Crown."

The Second Interception catches the low Middle and Underhews. The weapon is held diagonally downwards.

The Third Interception, against high Middle and Underhews, is the right outward-lying starting stance.

The Fourth Interception covers the left flank in the same way.

Any combinations of hew and interception are the Gliding Hews, whereby the opposing hew is deflected and, by gliding along the adversary's sword, one's own hew hits.

Ducking and Springing

A clever fencer can also evade the opposing hew by ducking a deep Middlehew or by springing away over a deep Underhew. Furthermore, the opposing attack can indeed be underrun during your advance; or you can spring directly towards the feet of the adversary, yet before his hew arrives, and "grip" him.

Grappling

Grappling is only allowed in the Forward Locus or as a last means of defense, when indeed only one foot is in your own locus. Grappling is only valid which disarms the adversary forthwith, throws him, or removes him from his locus. When the fencers begin to brawl, the fight-master breaks up the bout forthwith. When any adversary rests, for whatever reason, he is vanquished. There is to be no ground-struggle. Likewise, he has lost who becomes disarmed, disabled, or pushed out of the locus.

Invitation

The hesitant left fencer gets invited by exposure of the left side of the adversary, (striking) from this (hew) to a left hew, as illustrated.

The Fight-Master

To all proper fencing belongs a fight-master, who betters the fencer's stances; instructs his beginning, exiting, and conclusion; plus decides his hits, wins, and losses.

Hits suspend the bout only when the master orders *Halt!* But that is only needed in doubtful circumstances. Against the verdicts of the master, there are not any remonstrances while fencing. Afterwards, the bout can be reviewed.

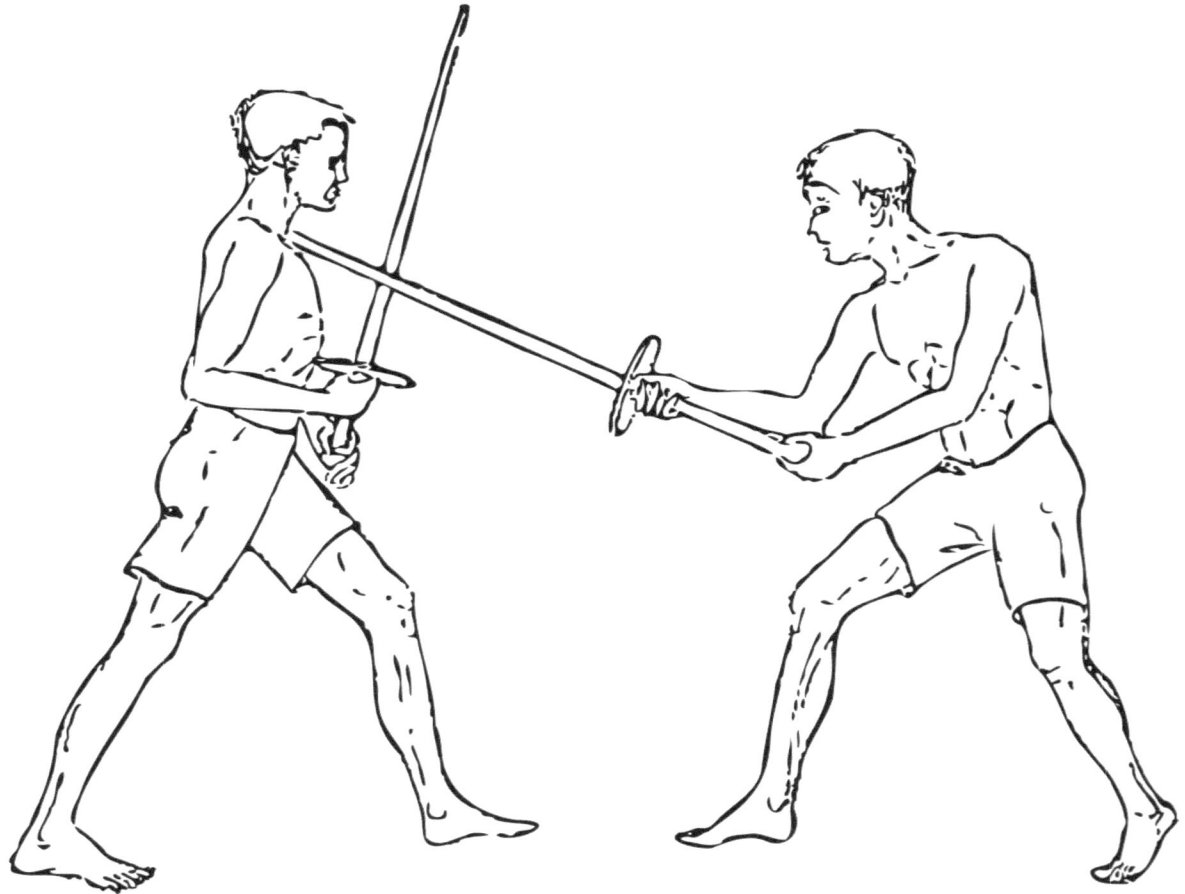

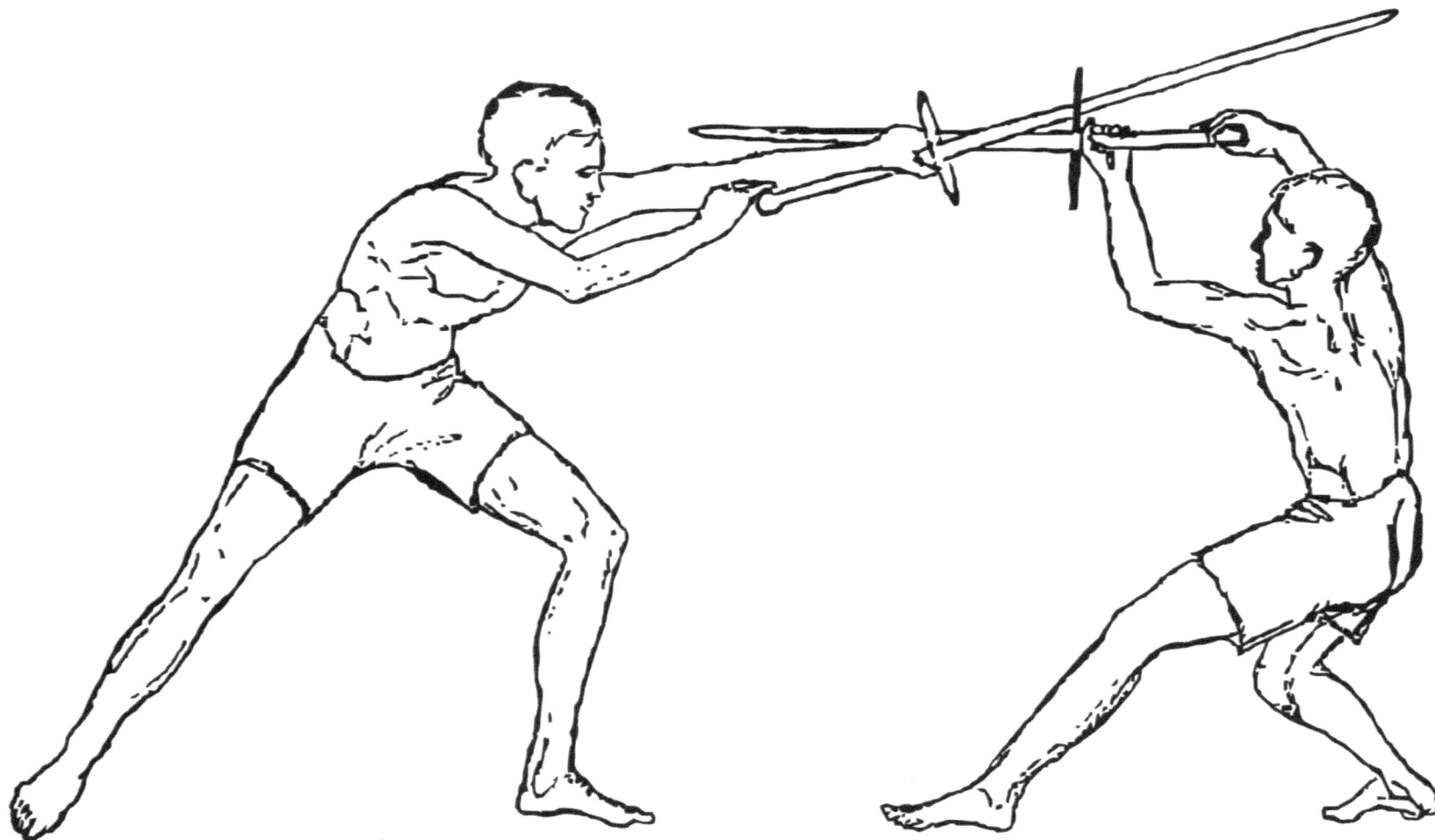

Entry — The left fencer attacks with wrath-hew. The right fencer diverts with first interception.

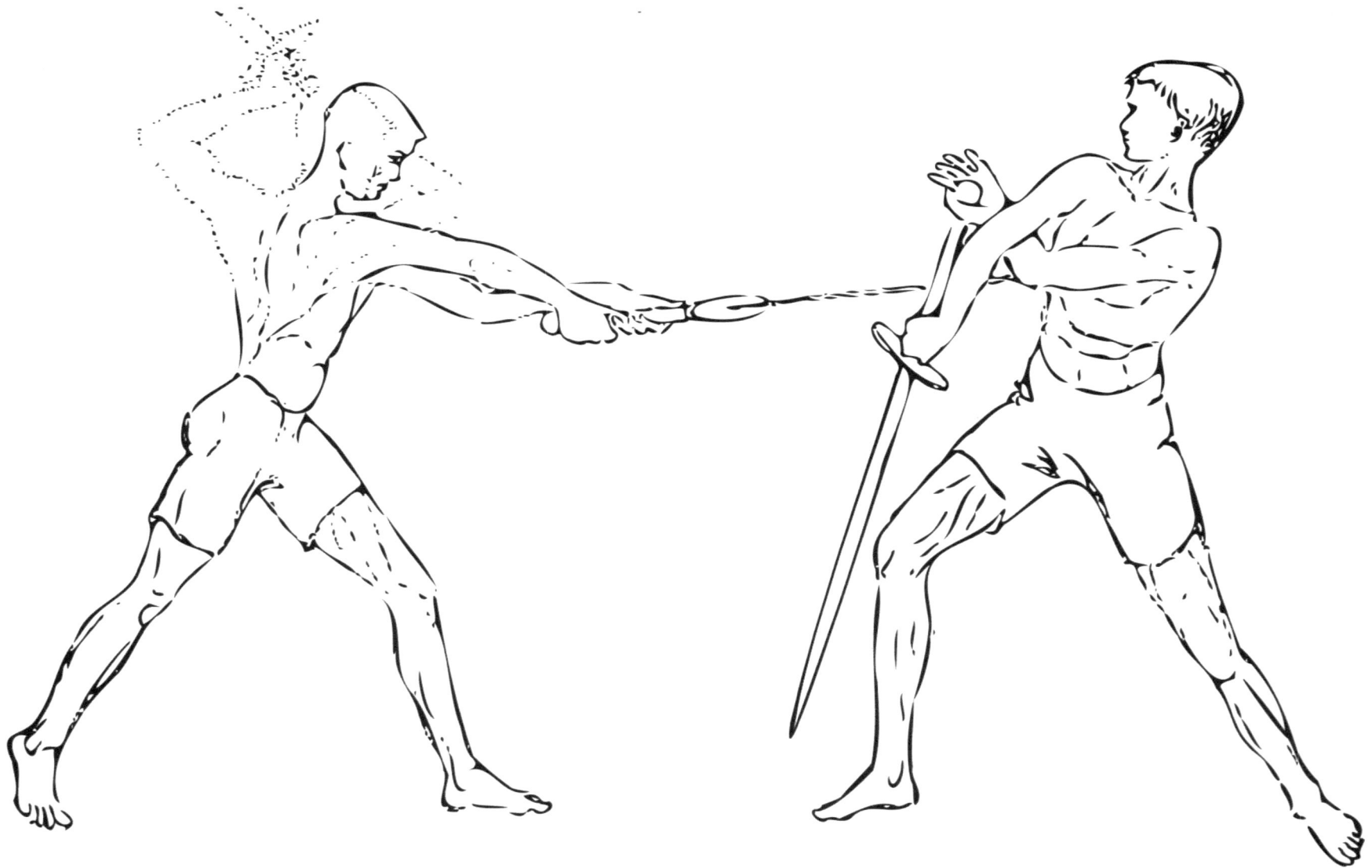

Entry – The left fencer attacks with right middlehew. The right fencer intercepts in the second interception with the hilt.

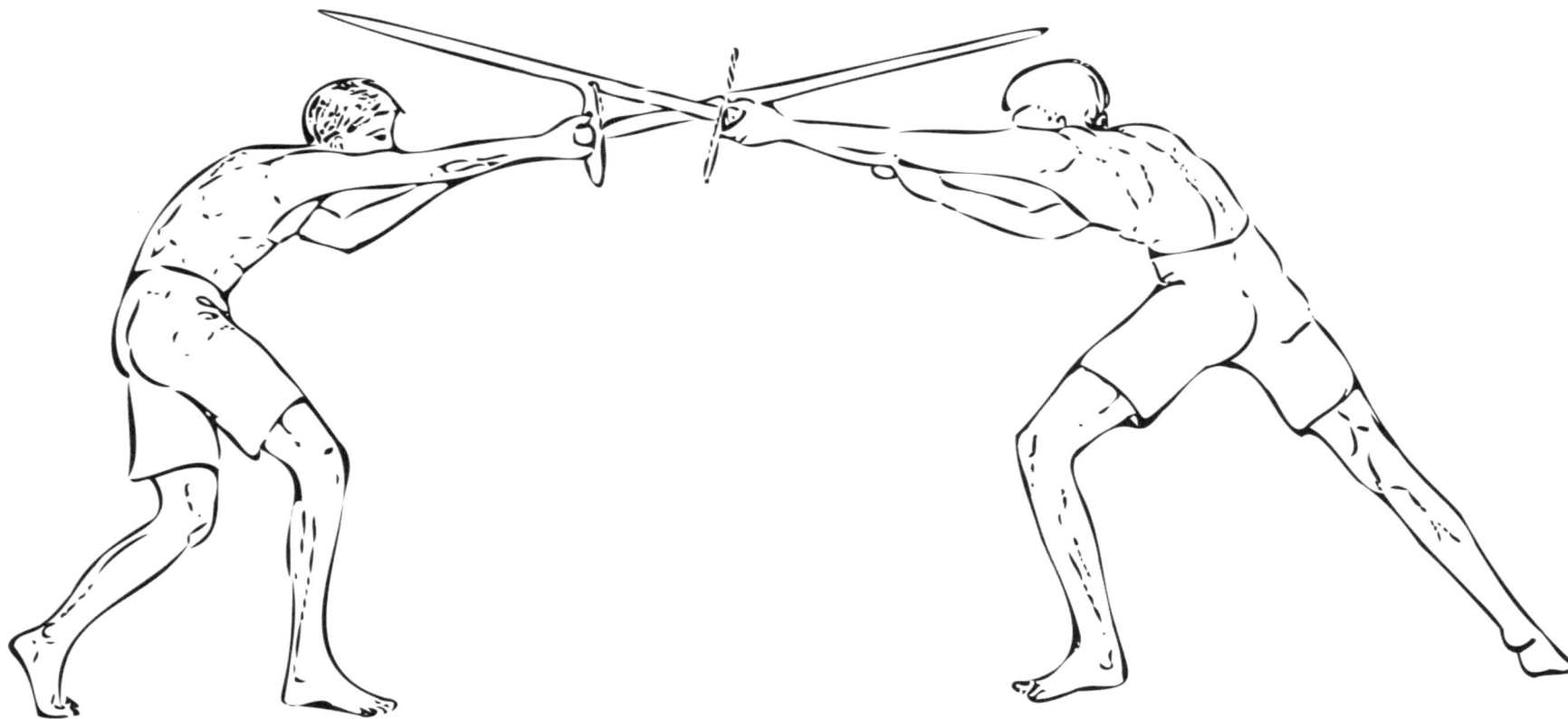

Entry – Hold all interceptions as far as possible from the body! Here the right fencer, a left-hander, attacks with a wrath-hew, which the left fencer diverts with the third interception. It is possible that the attacker himself thereby hews the sword of his adversary into his own right arm.

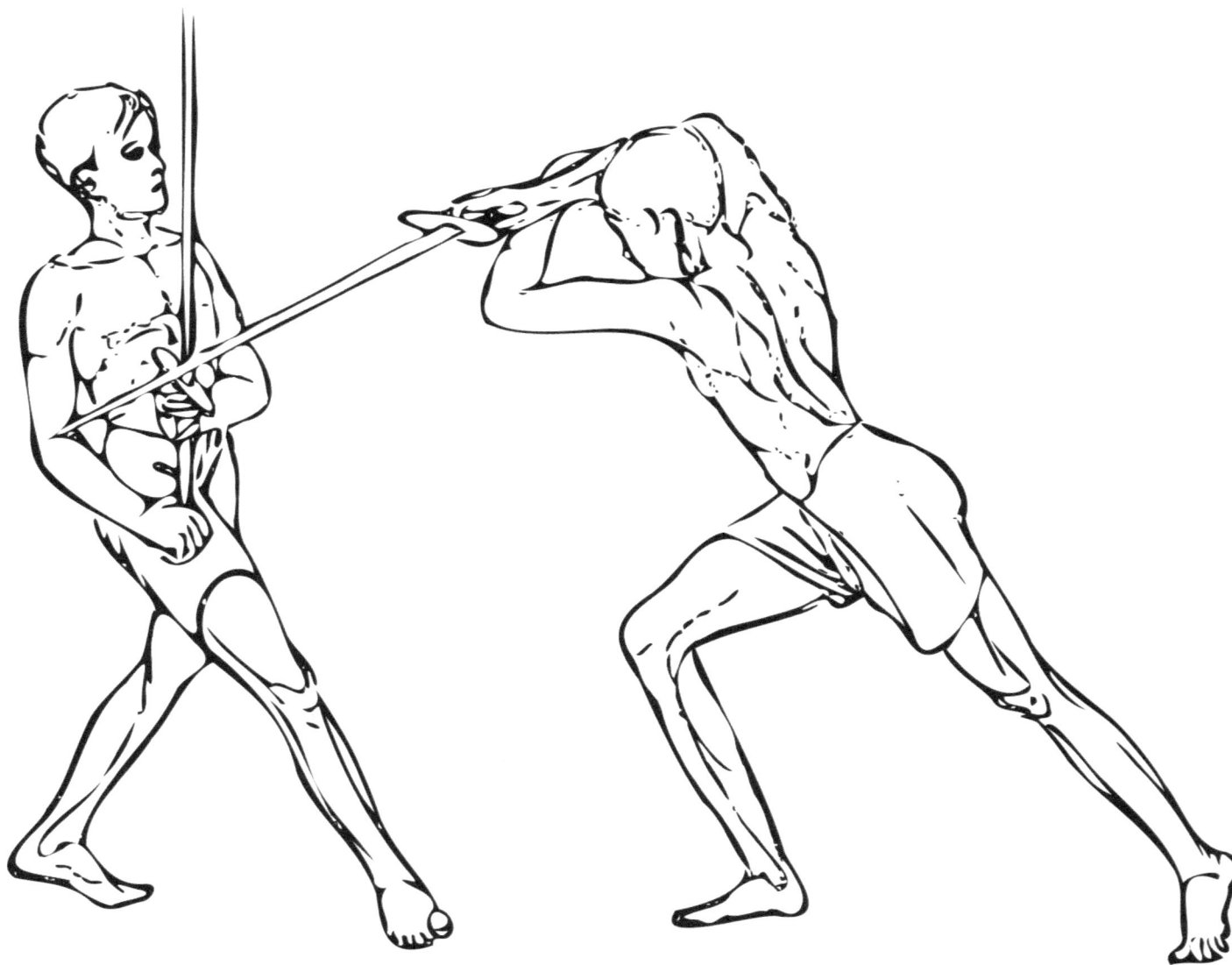

Counterstrike – The right fencer speeds an underhew from the second interception as counterstrike, which the adversary diverts with one step backwards into the fourth interception.

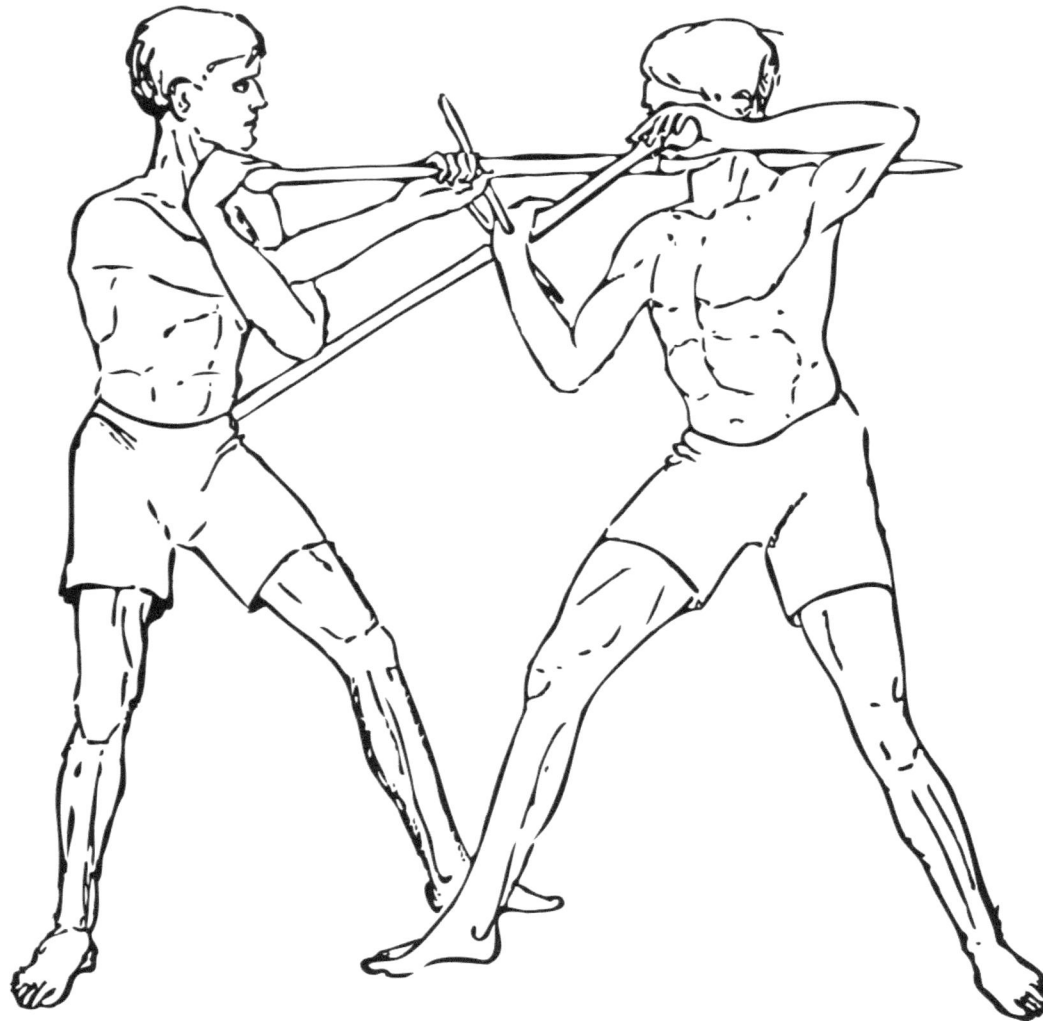

Engagement – The right fencer attacks with underhew up to the left fencer's elbow. The adversary counters the hew through right twisted overhew with the strong and hits the attacker synchronously with the weak to the neck.

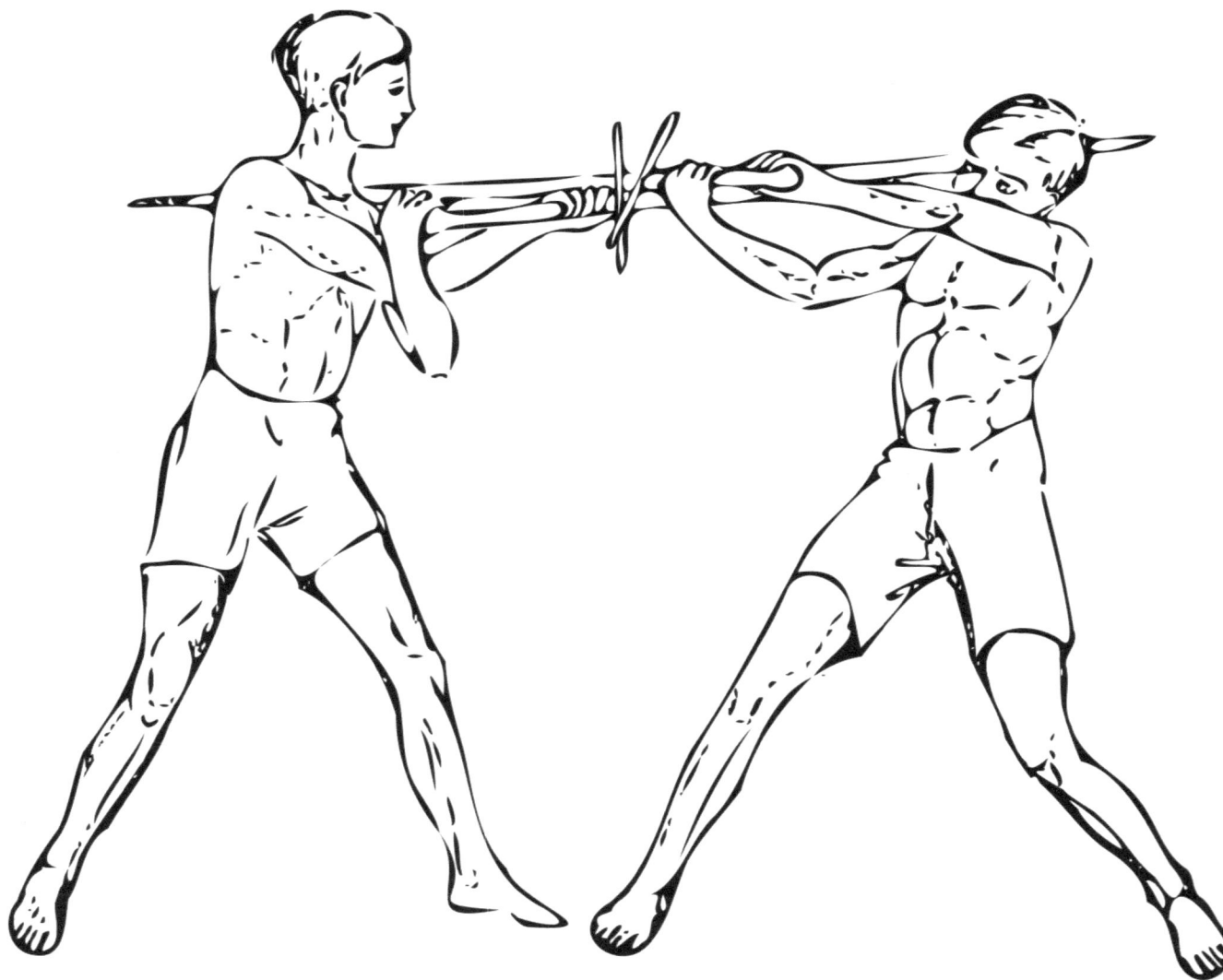

Glide-Hew – A right middlehew by the right fencer gets countered by a far-forward-placed glide-hew by the adversary. The sword glides along at the weapon of the attacker, strikes it aside and hits him upon the head.

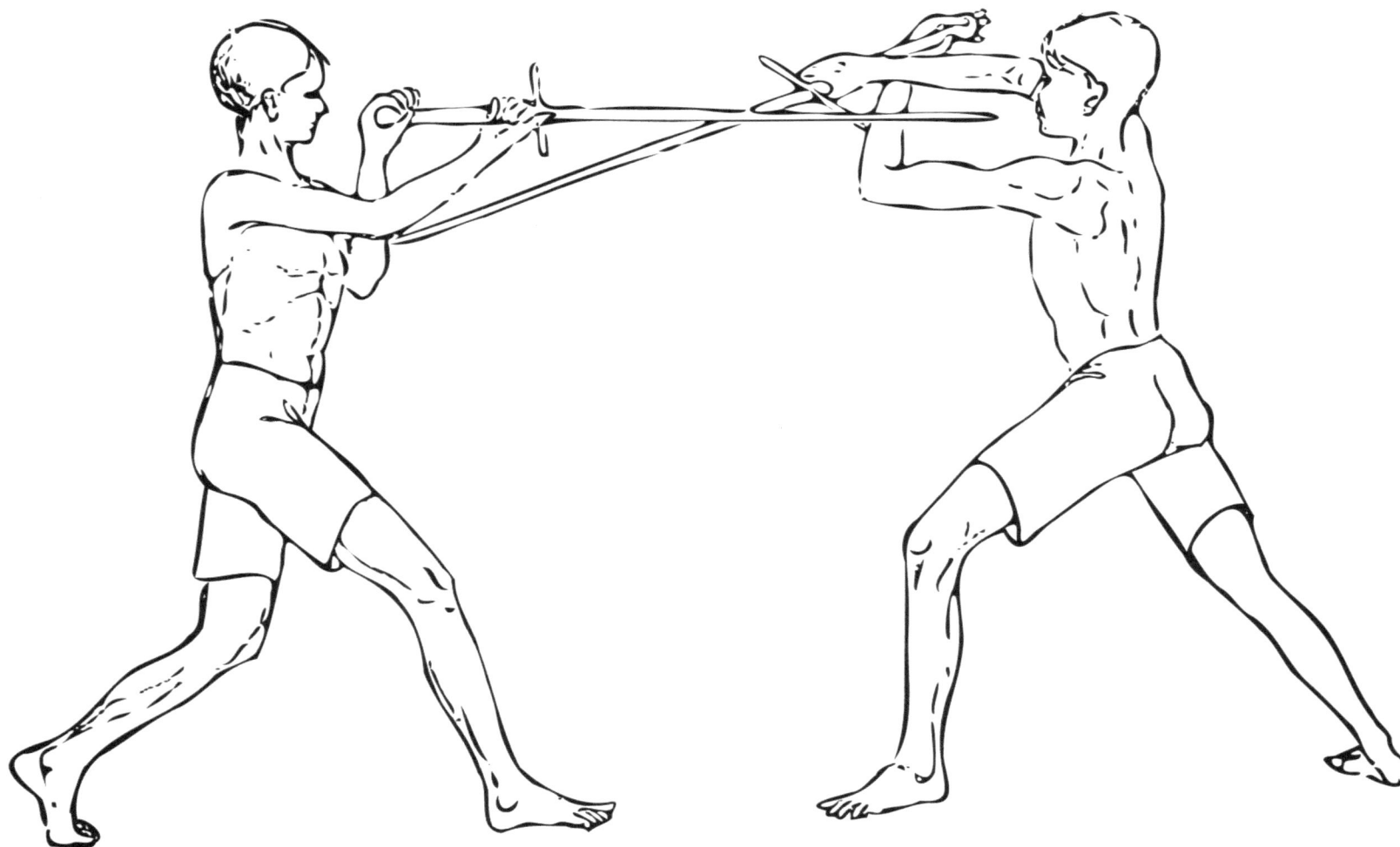

Engagement – A bout taken from Dürer's fight-book[14]: The left fencer attacks with left underhew. The adversary strikes an underhew against that, which upwardly "parries/excludes" the sword of the attacker. Thereby he hits the elbow. This defense is very effective, but requires great velocity, otherwise a hit under one's own left arm is unavoidable.

---

[14] Longsword Action 12

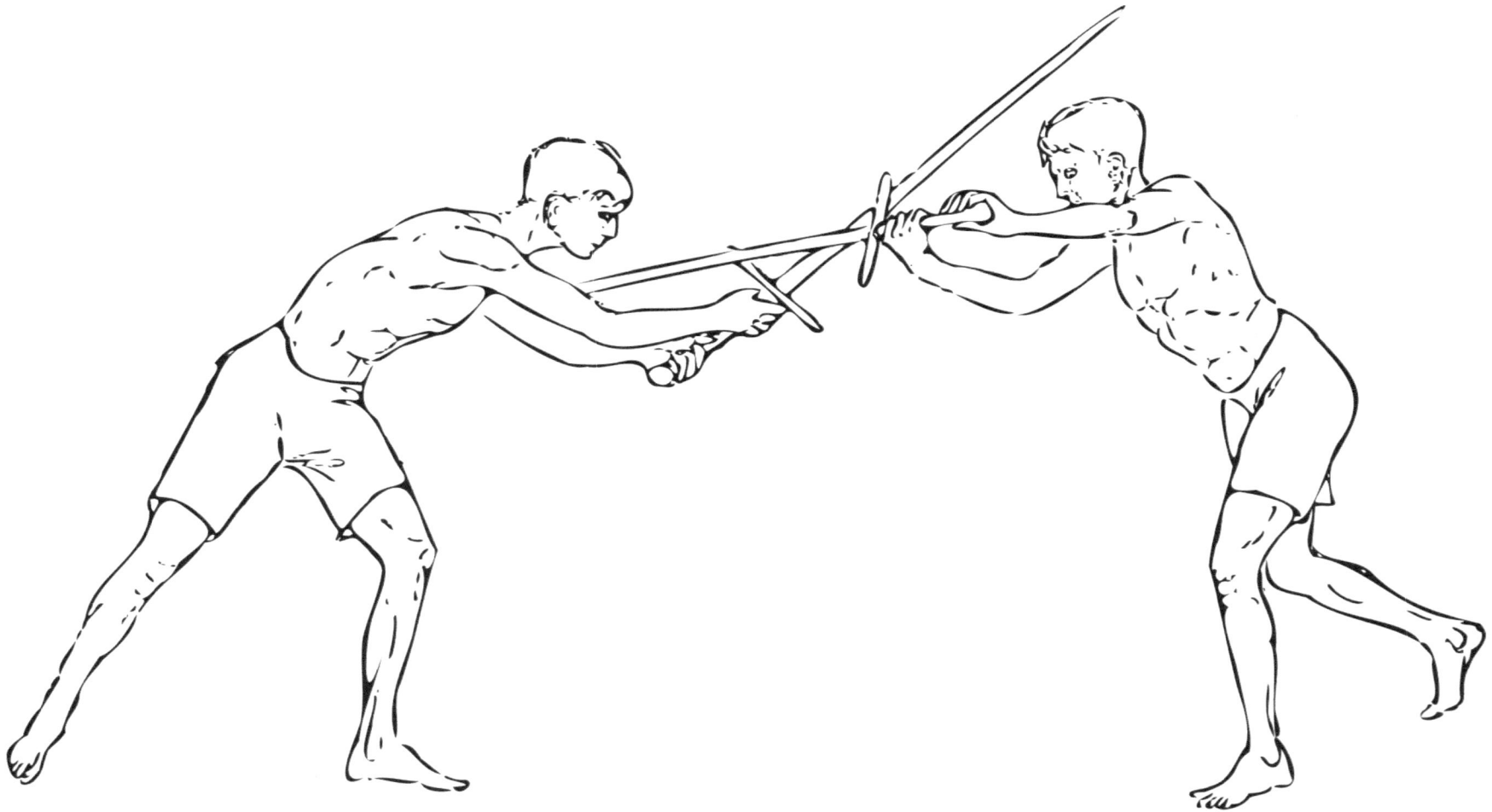

Exit — The right fencer parries a wrath-hew by the adversary towards the right. A left middlehew as countercut must hit.

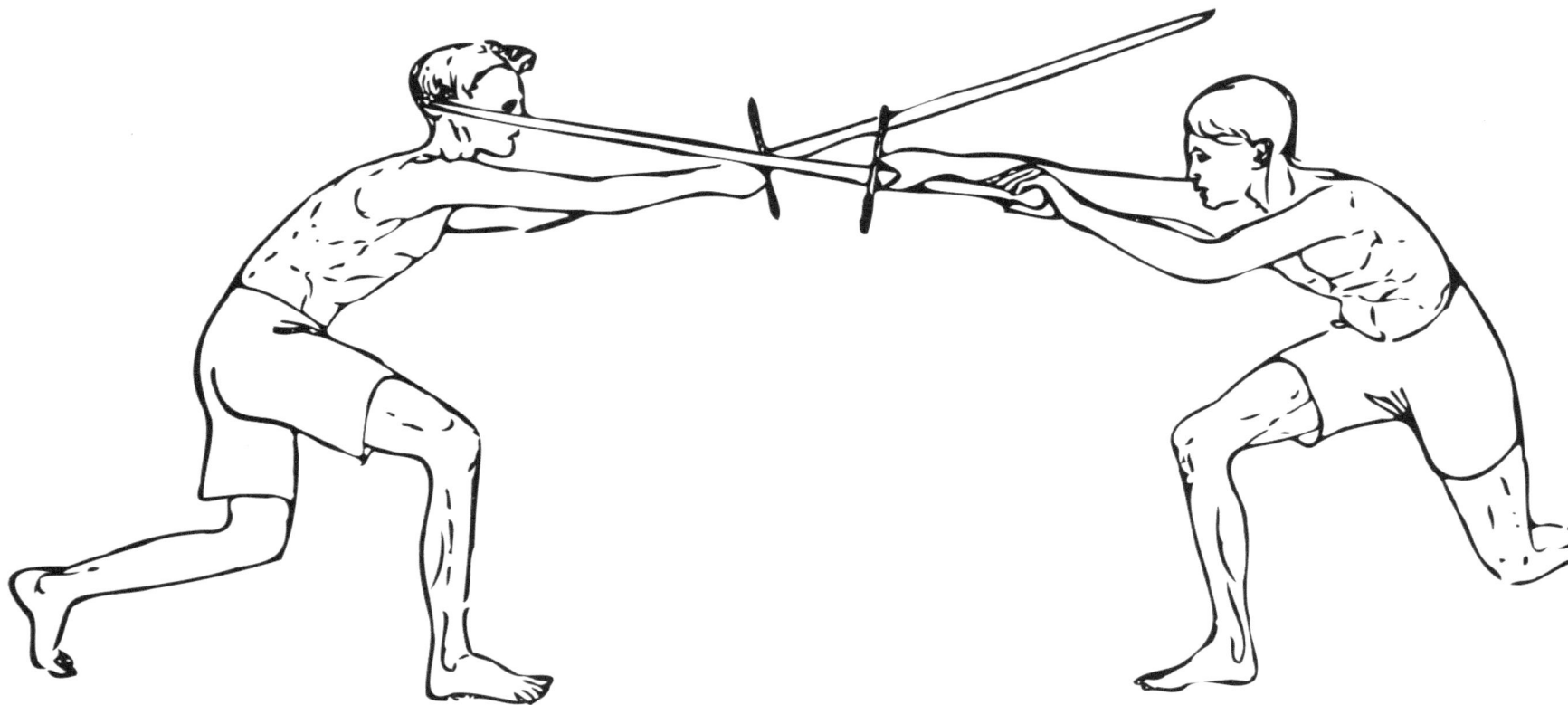

Exit: "Bounce-Hew"/"Cheat-Hew" — The right fencer evades an opposing right overhew by ducking. The hew goes over him and away. He hits synchronously with the flat of the blade ("bouncehew"/"cheat-hew") to the adversary's head.

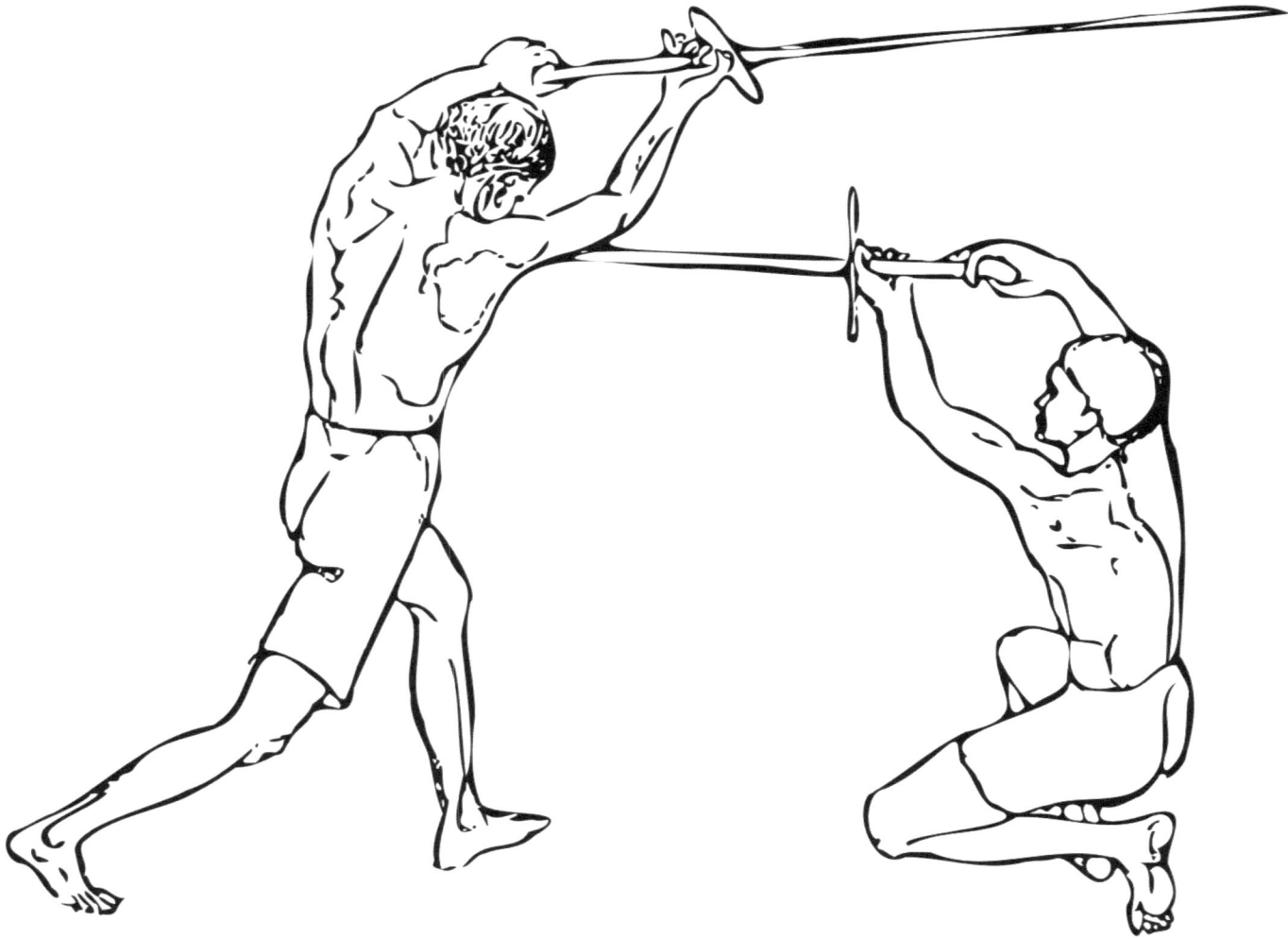

Exit: Ducking – The right fencer evades a high middlehew by kneeling/squatting and synchronously strikes an underhew, which hits.

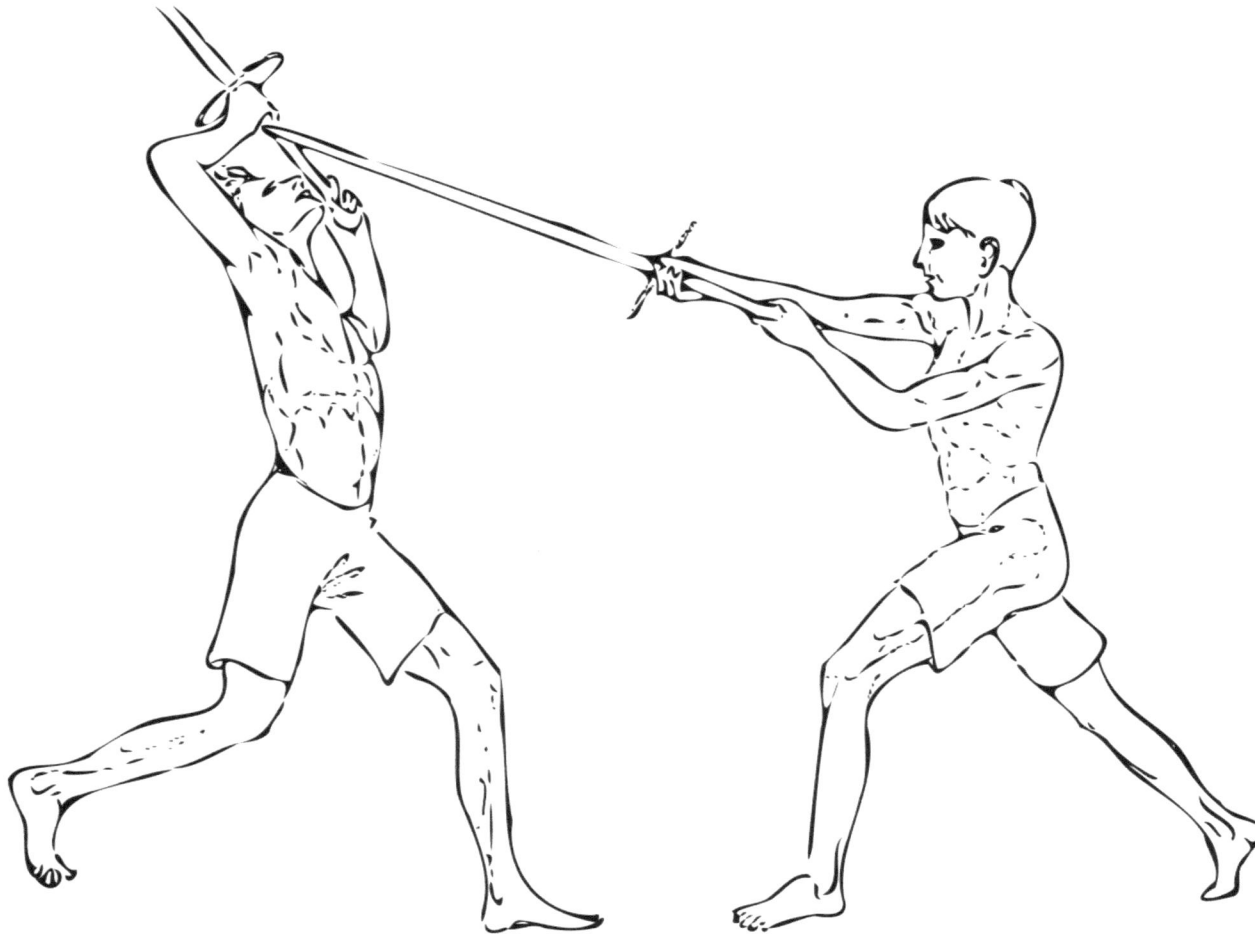

Entry or Exit: "Hew Inthereof" – The left fencer attacks too hastily with a "hew From the Day." The right fencer goes at him with a "hew inthereof" and hits earlier. This hew is only valid, if it were accelerated at least 1/4 of a circular arc. There are not to be collisions[15] in our fencing, because of the injuries which tend to happen therefrom.

---

[15] Consider the routinely injurious collisions of modern HEMA tourneys; injurious despite the massive and expensive safety gear worn by the adult fencers; thus evincing circa 2017 "martial artists" cannot bring themselves to respect their peers and control their strikes like circa 1935 German kids evidently strove to do.

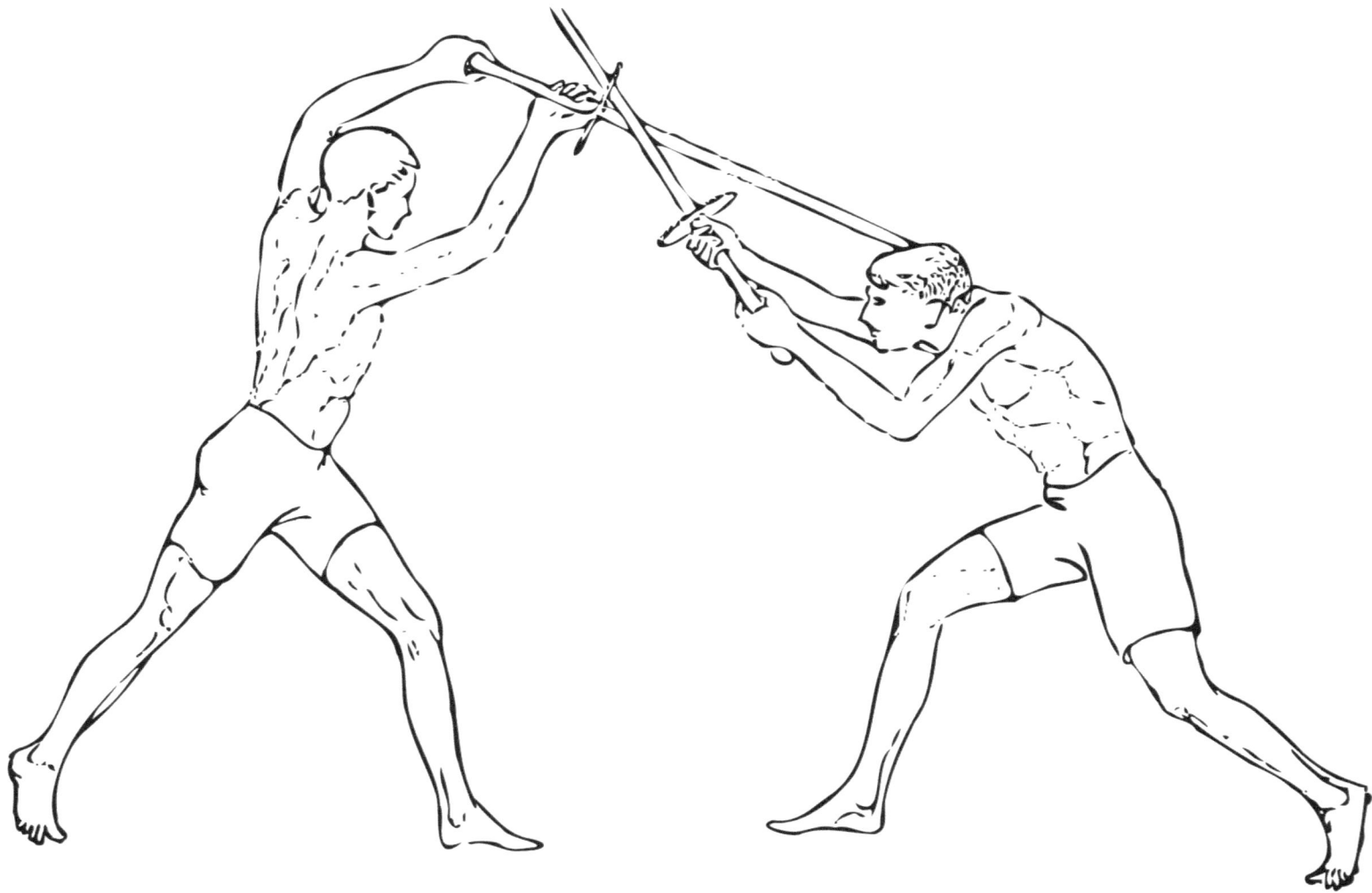

The "Masterly Squint-Hew" — One good play / action for great fencers. The left fencer wards off a wrath-hew by the adversary in the first interception and spins himself thereby, so that the adversary injures himself.

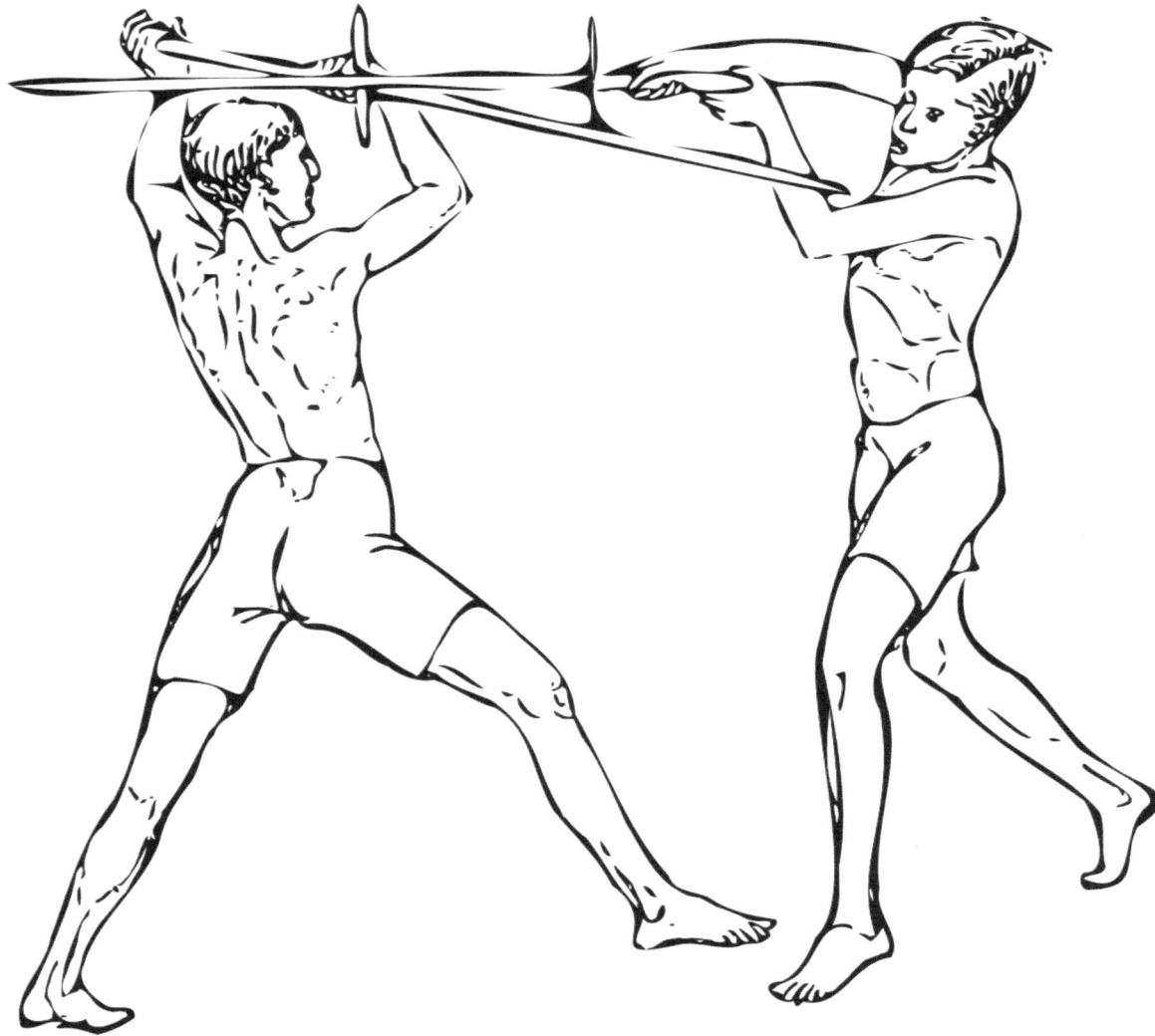

The "Minor Squint-Hew" — is for fencers who fight with great adversaries. Also here is an interception like in the first situation (Glide-Hew pg. 18 or Engagement pg. 19), whereby the attacker strikes the opposing sword into his arm.

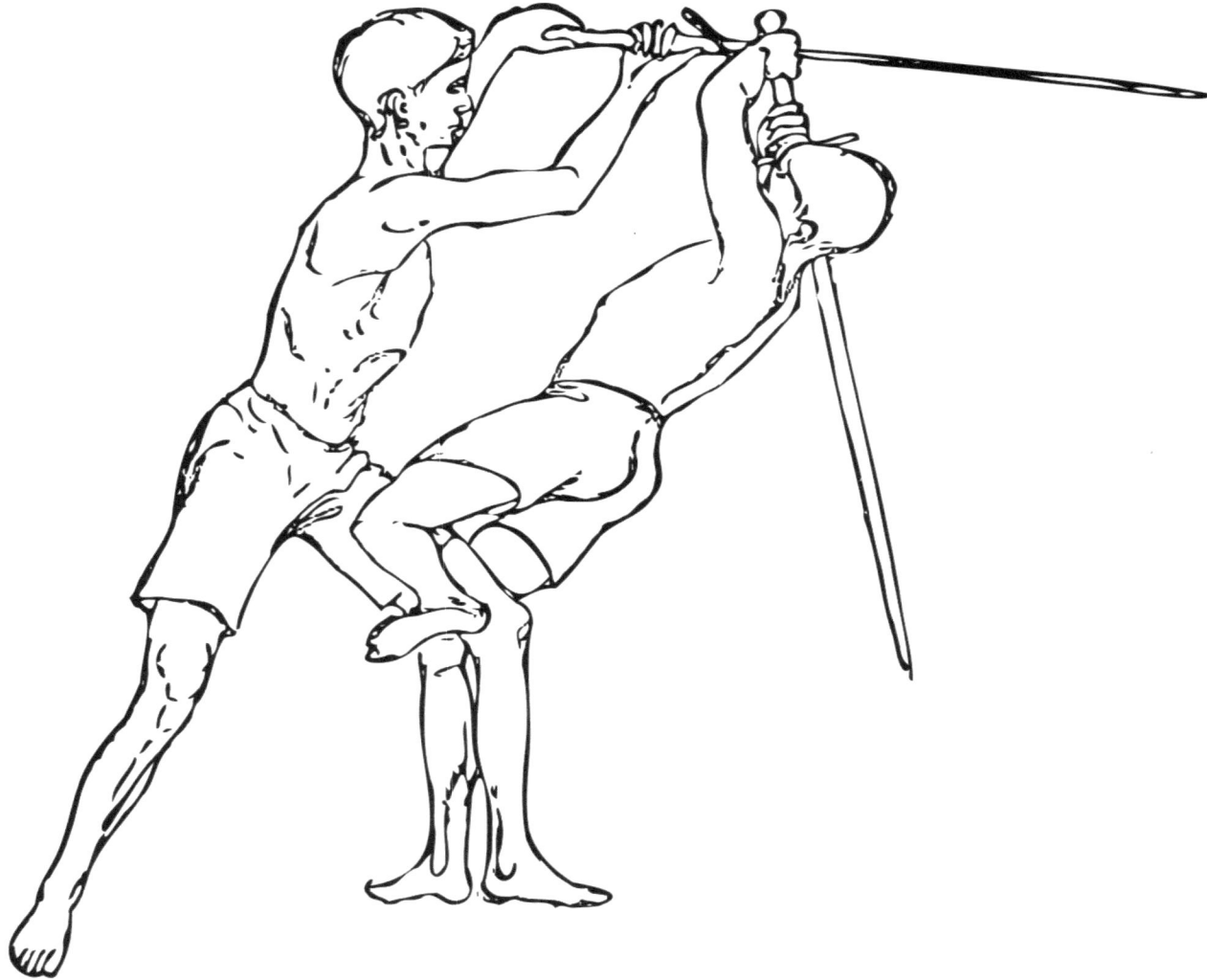

"Feeling Inthereof" — The left fencer catches an opposing wrath-hew already during advancement, and either throws the weak adversary upon his back by sharp riposte with the cross, or takes the strong adversary's sword from him.

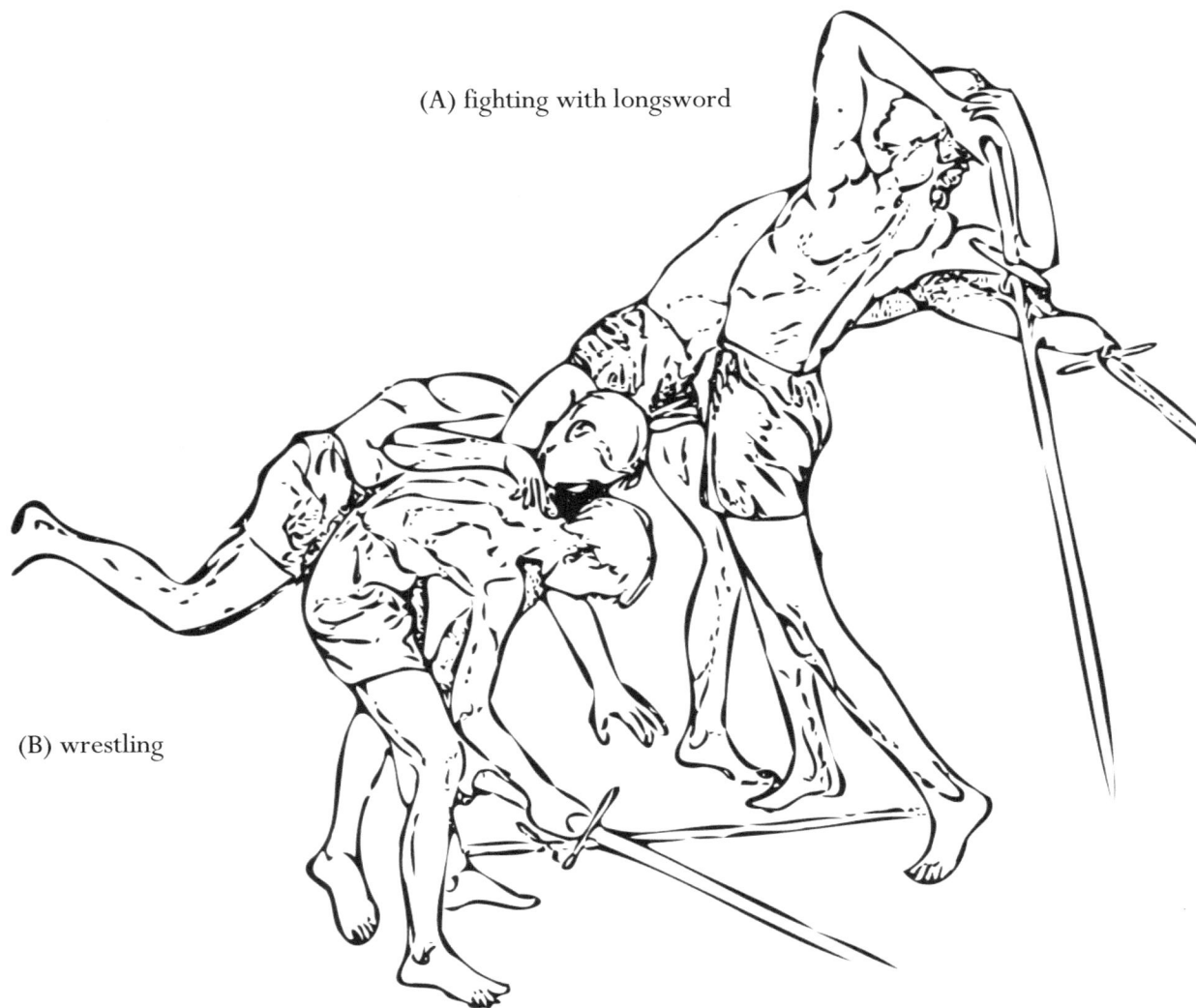

(A) fighting with longsword

(B) wrestling

Counterward to the "Feeling Inthereof" – (A) The attacked (right fencer) evades the riposte, wherein he—supported from behind by his sword—spins himself swiftly right. Thereby he releases his left arm and (B) wraps it around the neck of the tumbling-past adversary and throws him via hip-toss.

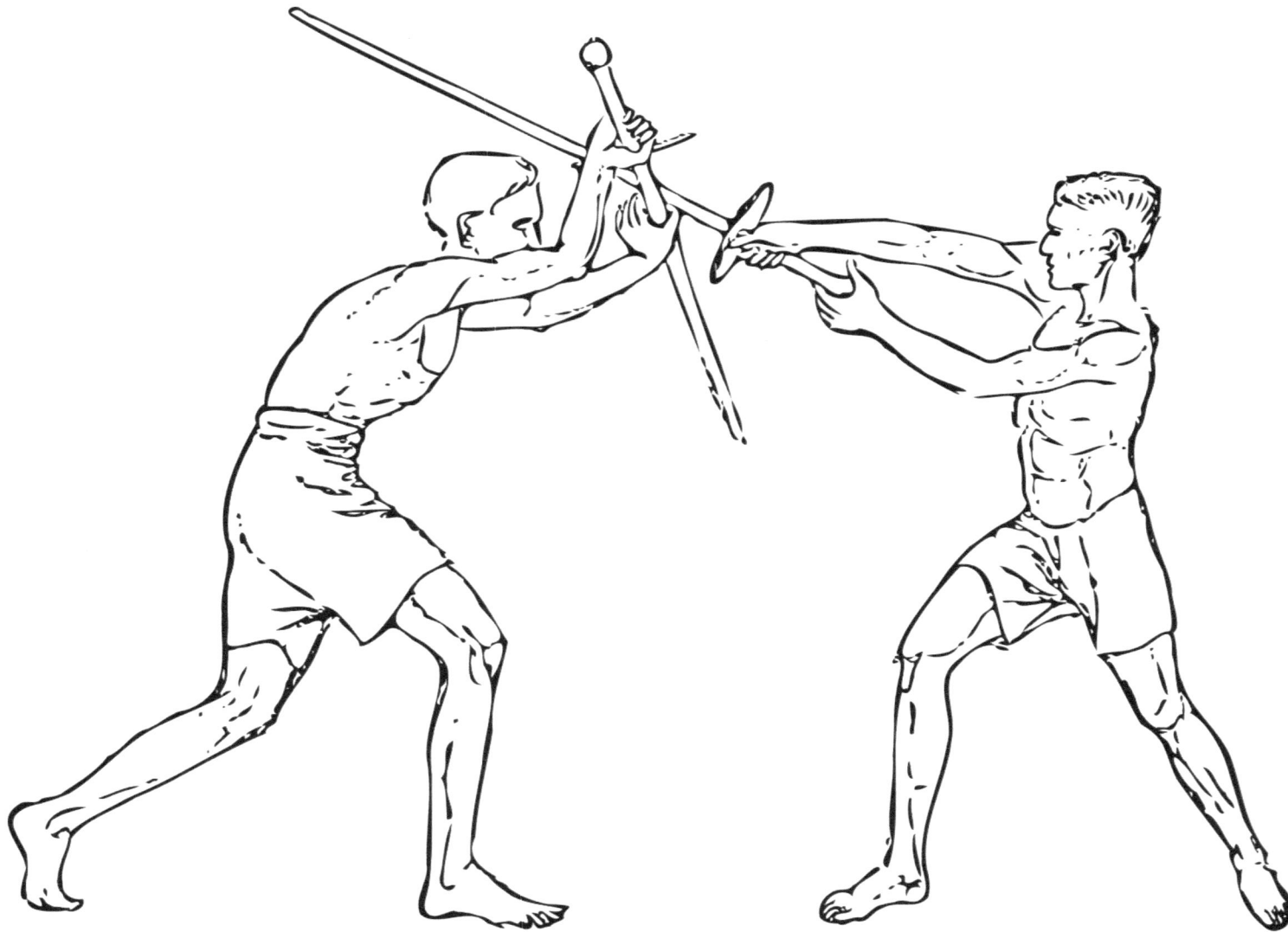

"The Crown" – The left fencer intercepts an opposing wrath-hew with the crown. Anyone who puts the edge instead of the flat in the hand while doing this is effectively hit.

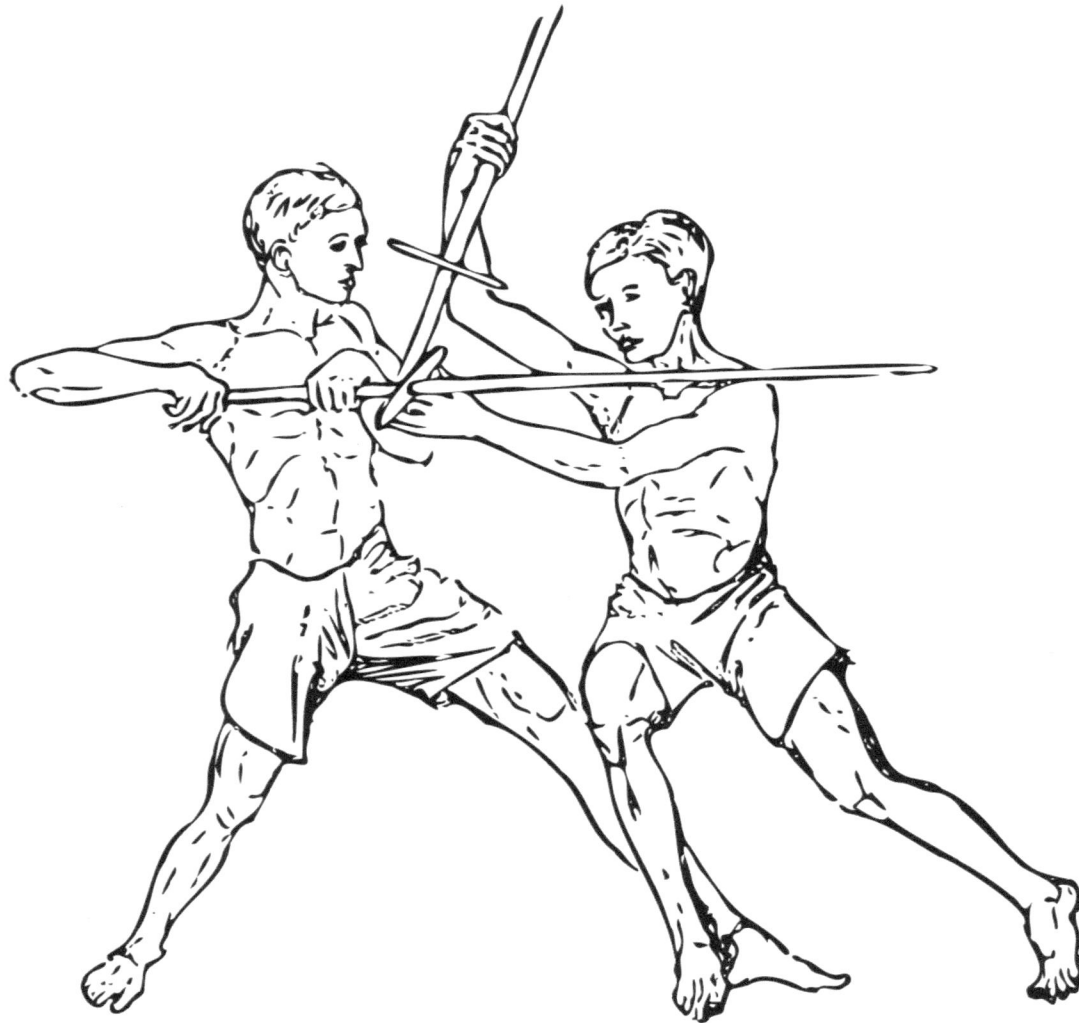

"A good move for an agile man" — The left fencer makes a wide left step forwards from the "crown," puts the weak of his sword at the left side of the adversary's throat, and pulls him over the widely outstretched leg. He takes the adversary's sword and brings him to fall.

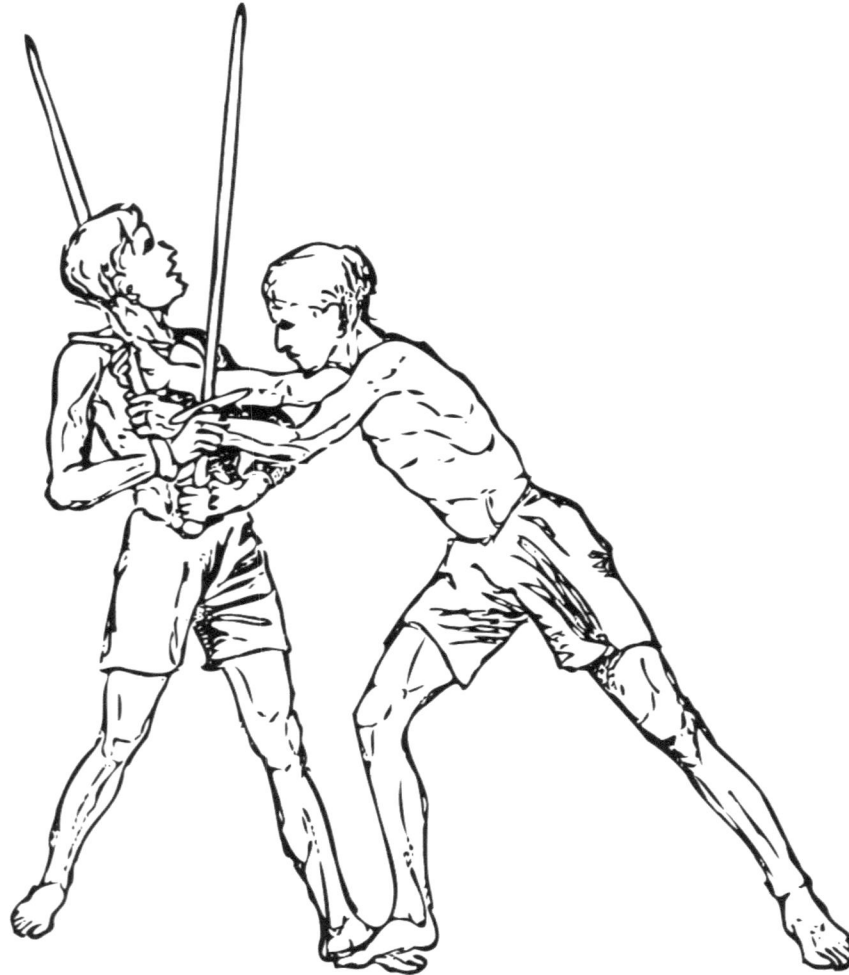

"A masterly move for every strong and agile man" — So you have hewn at the elbow of someone and he intercepts the hew, so push him down by the hilt of his sword and drop upon him with pommel and both arms and put your short edge at his throat as you step upon his foot—as illustrated here—and pull him so that you take his sword from him. [16]

---

[16] From the Meyer fencing manuscript circa 1600.

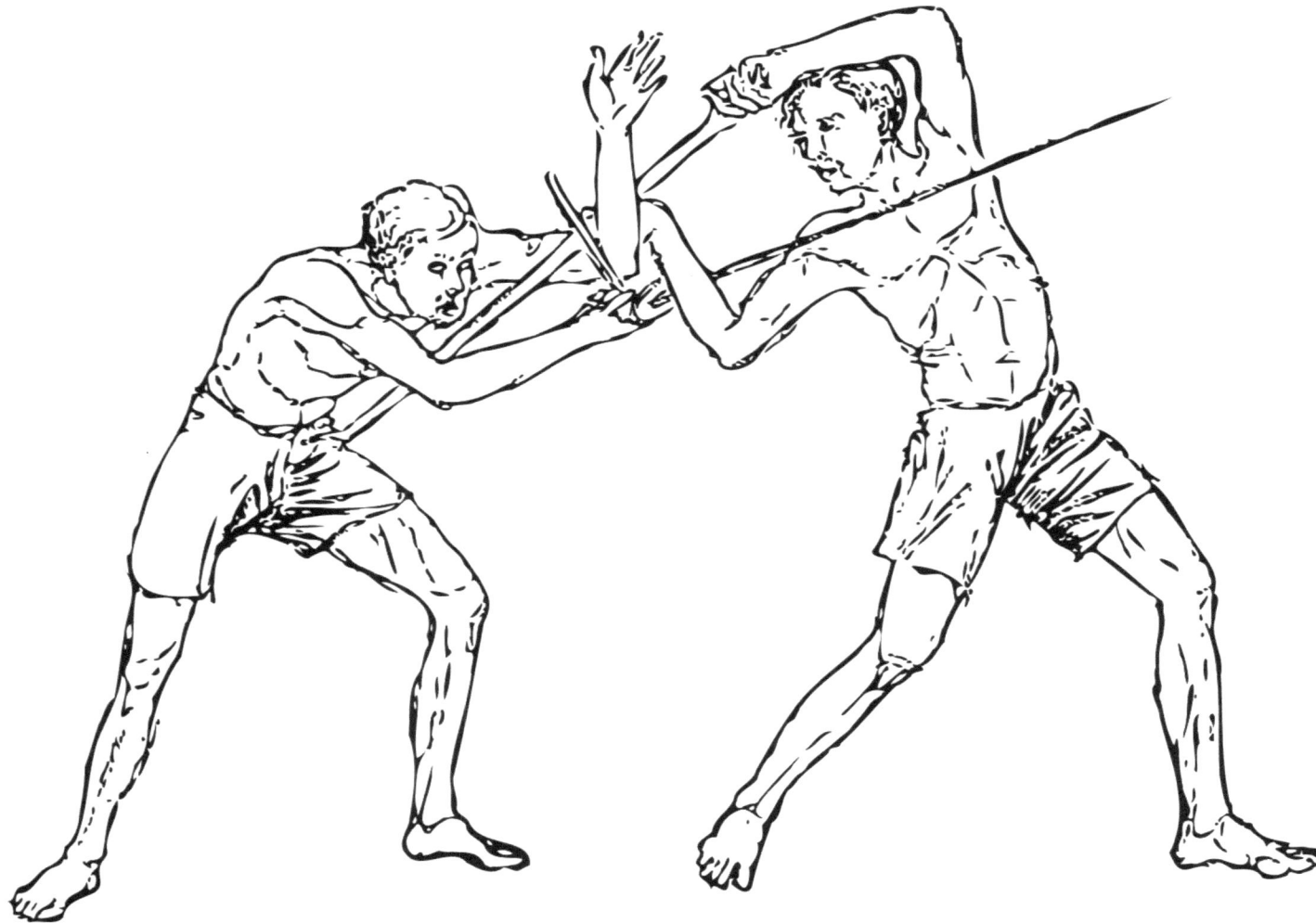

Another "Master-Move" — A fail-hew (feint) by the left fencer gets the adversary to do a second interception. The attacker releases his left hand from his sword and catches the weapon of the adversary from beneath and behind the cross with the left elbow-joint. Then he shoves through his sword between the right arm and the throat of the adversary. "So thou breakest his arm, so thou slittest his throat."

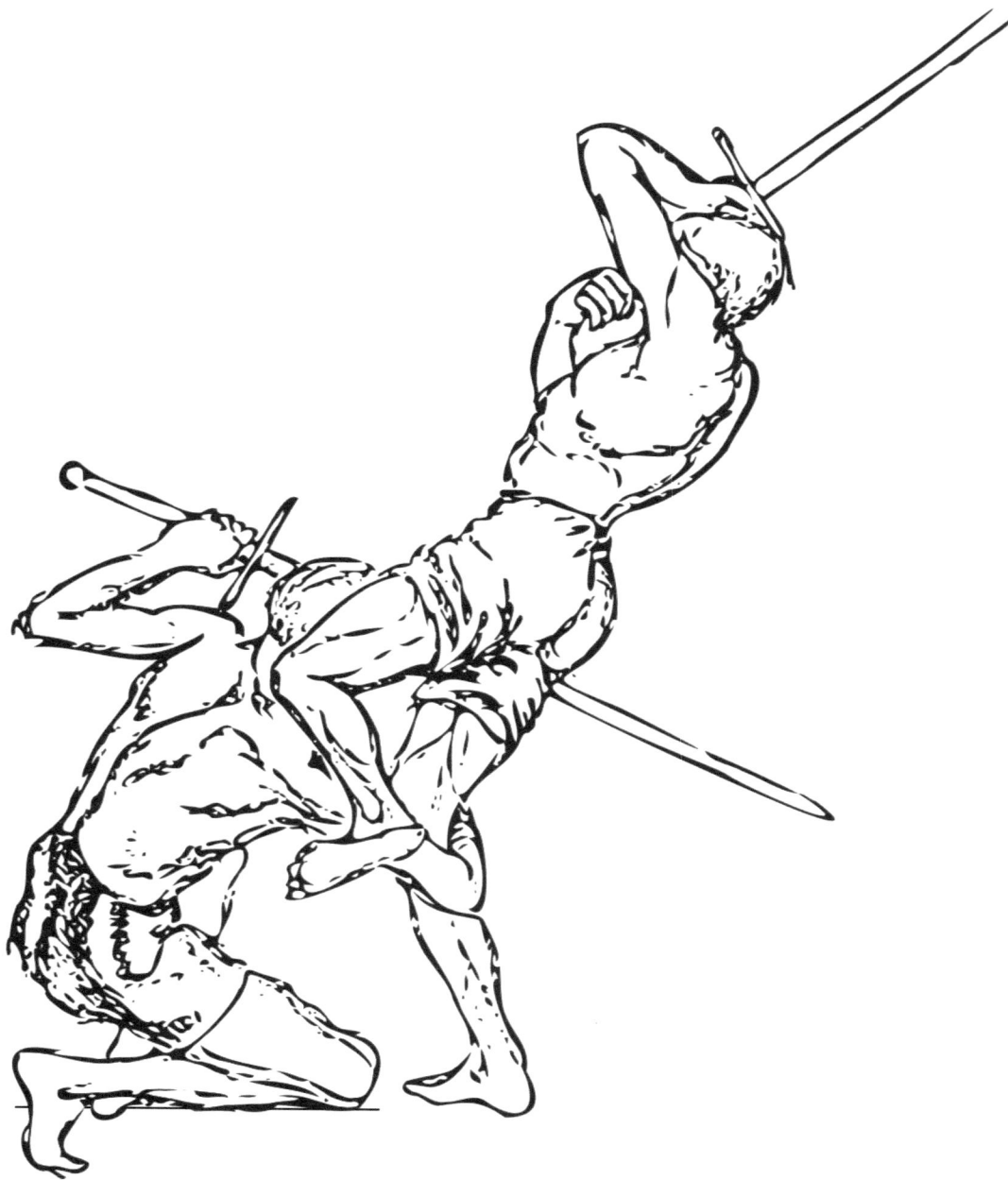

Grappling: Also a Master-Move – "So someone is slowly into advancement and will hew From the Day, so be agile and let thy sword fall and seize him quickly at the knee, heave him and press thy head against him, thus thou throwest him upon his back. That is one good play for any strong and agile man."[17]

---

[17] From the Meyer fight-book circa 1600.

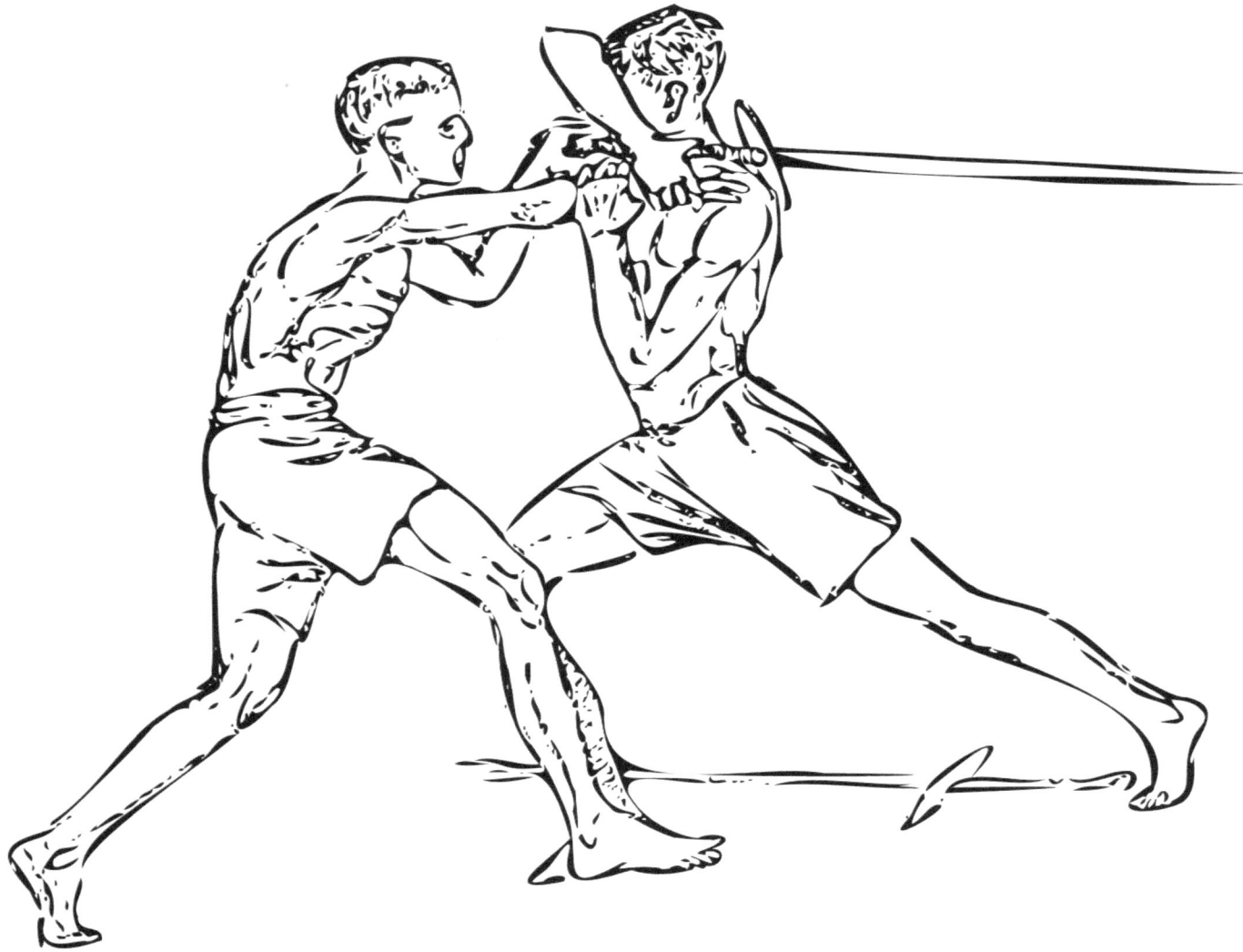

"Intrusion" 1 — The right fencer underruns a wrath-hew by the adversary. The left hand seizes the opposing right hand from beneath at the wrist while the right hand seizes over the backhand from above. Then the seized hand gets spun around quickly to the right.

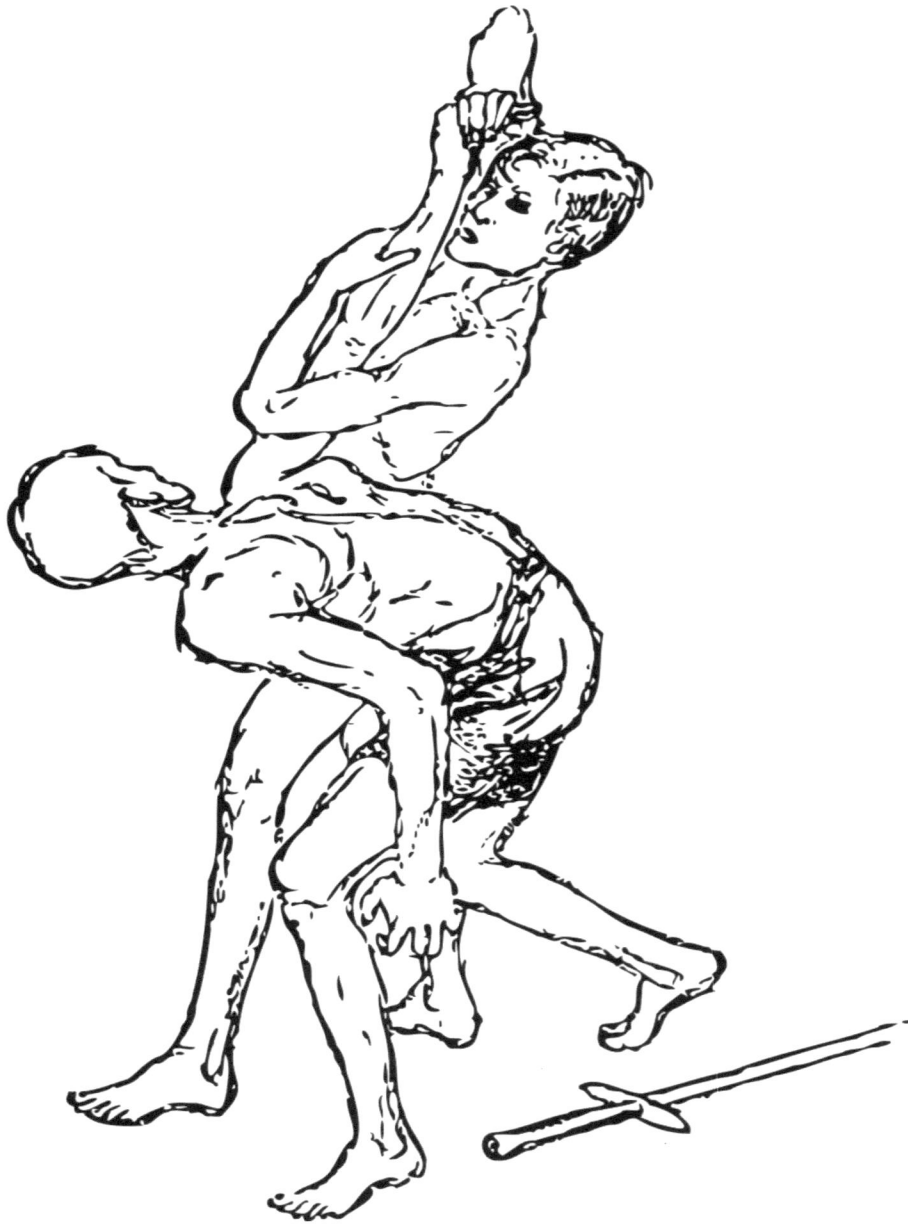

"Intrusion" 2 — Pull the seized arm of the adversary under and through your left arm and press his wrist downwards. The adversary is helpless.

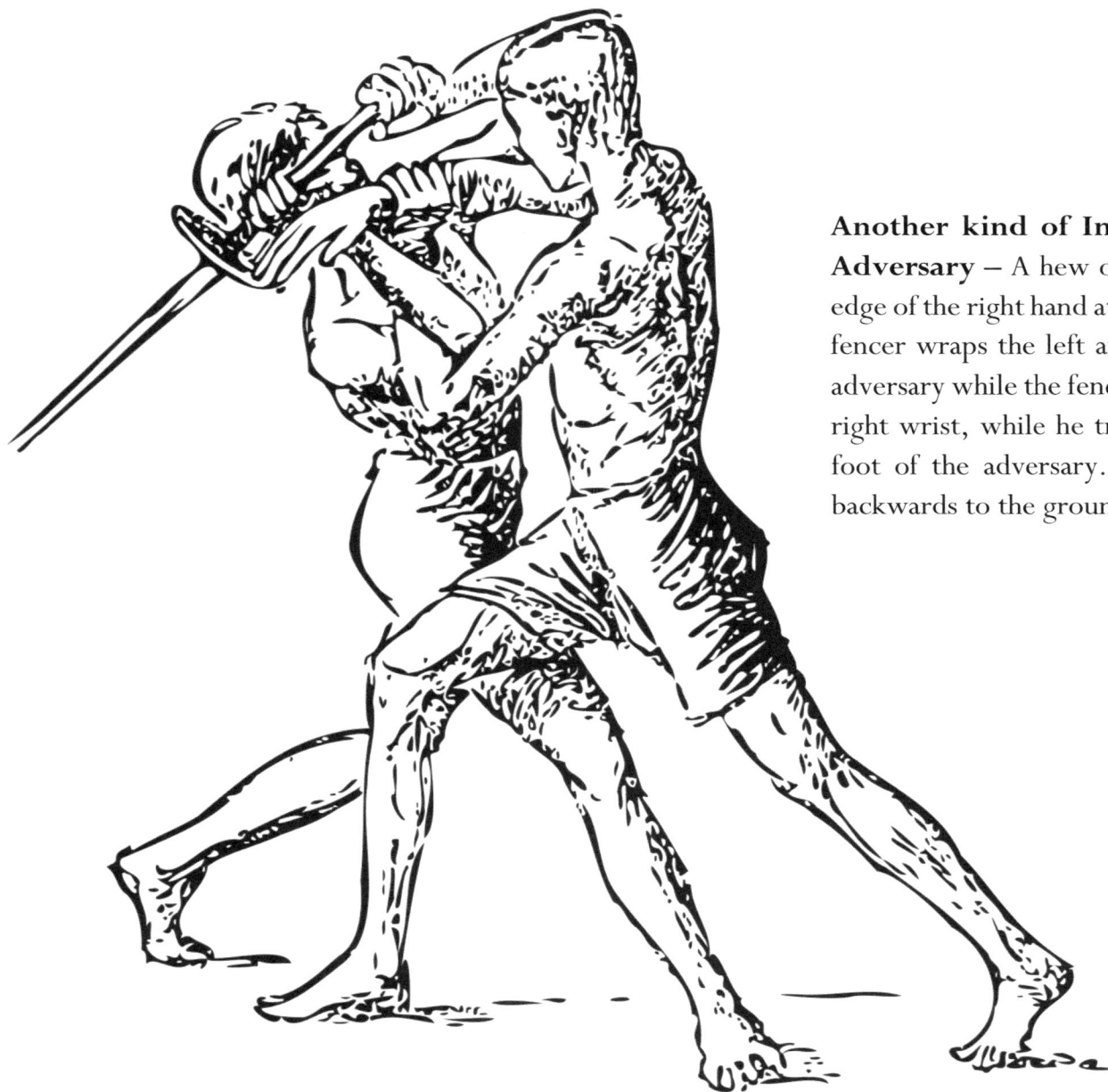

Another kind of Intrusion (3), which throws the Adversary – A hew of the adversary gets caught with the edge of the right hand at the right wrist of the adversary. The fencer wraps the left arm into the right elbow joint of the adversary while the fencer's left hand holds fast onto his own right wrist, while he treads the right foot behind the right foot of the adversary. Now you can press the adversary backwards to the ground.

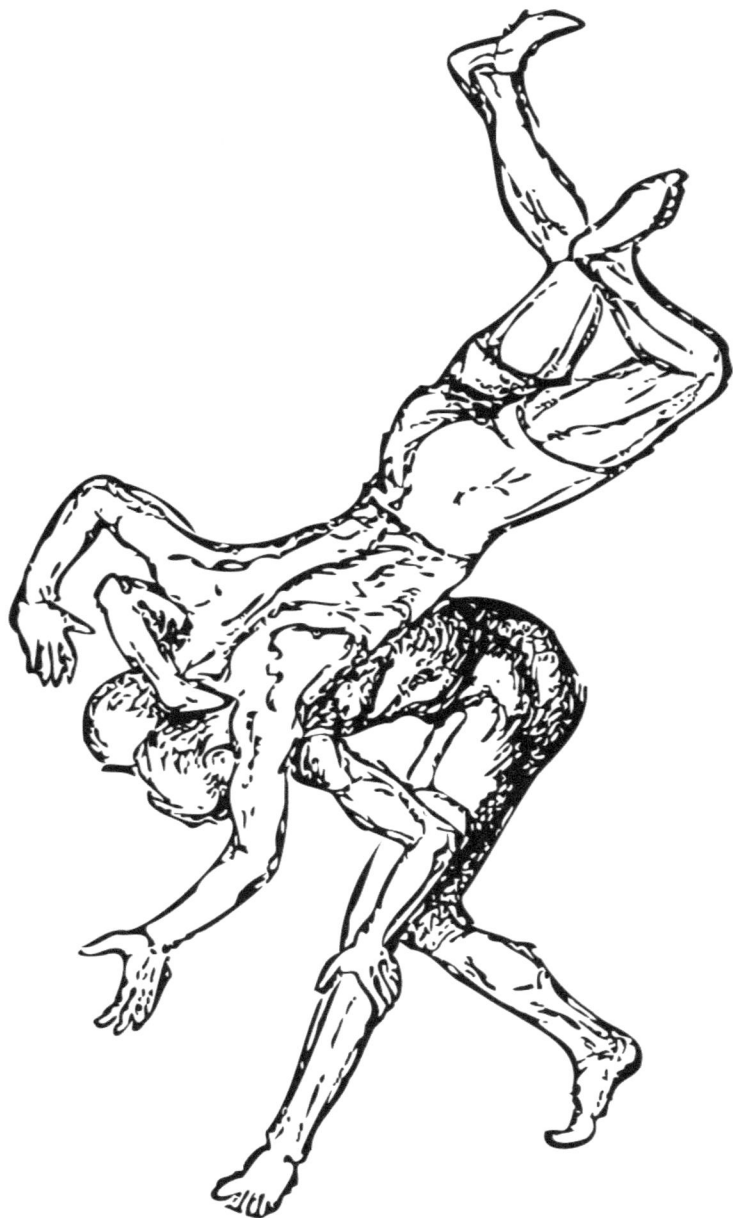

Throwing via Shoulder-Toss — When the adversary has "intruded" you, then spring immediately before him, make a sharp turn and thereby wrap your arm around his neck—as illustrated here—thus you can throw him over your shoulder and overhead to the ground. During the performance: The attacker must let loose punctually—thus neither too early nor too late! The thrown fencer comes down upon his feet when he makes the sacrum of his back rather concave while somersaulting himself!

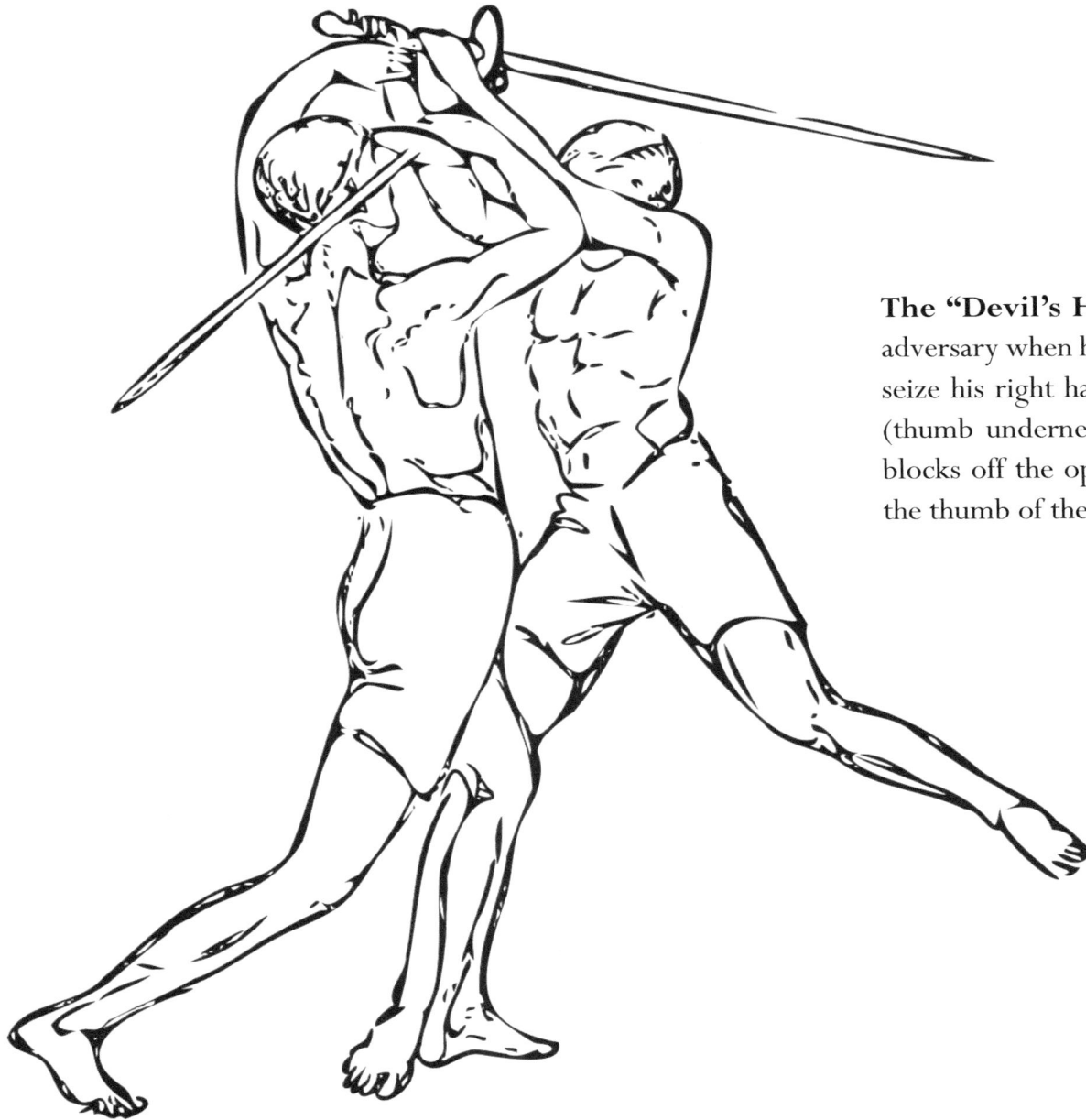

The "Devil's Handshake" — If you are intruding the adversary when he will hew From the Day, then inthereof seize his right hand with your left hand in standard grip (thumb underneath and outside) while your right hand blocks off the opposing left hand (with your hilt); press the thumb of the adversary fast against his little finger…

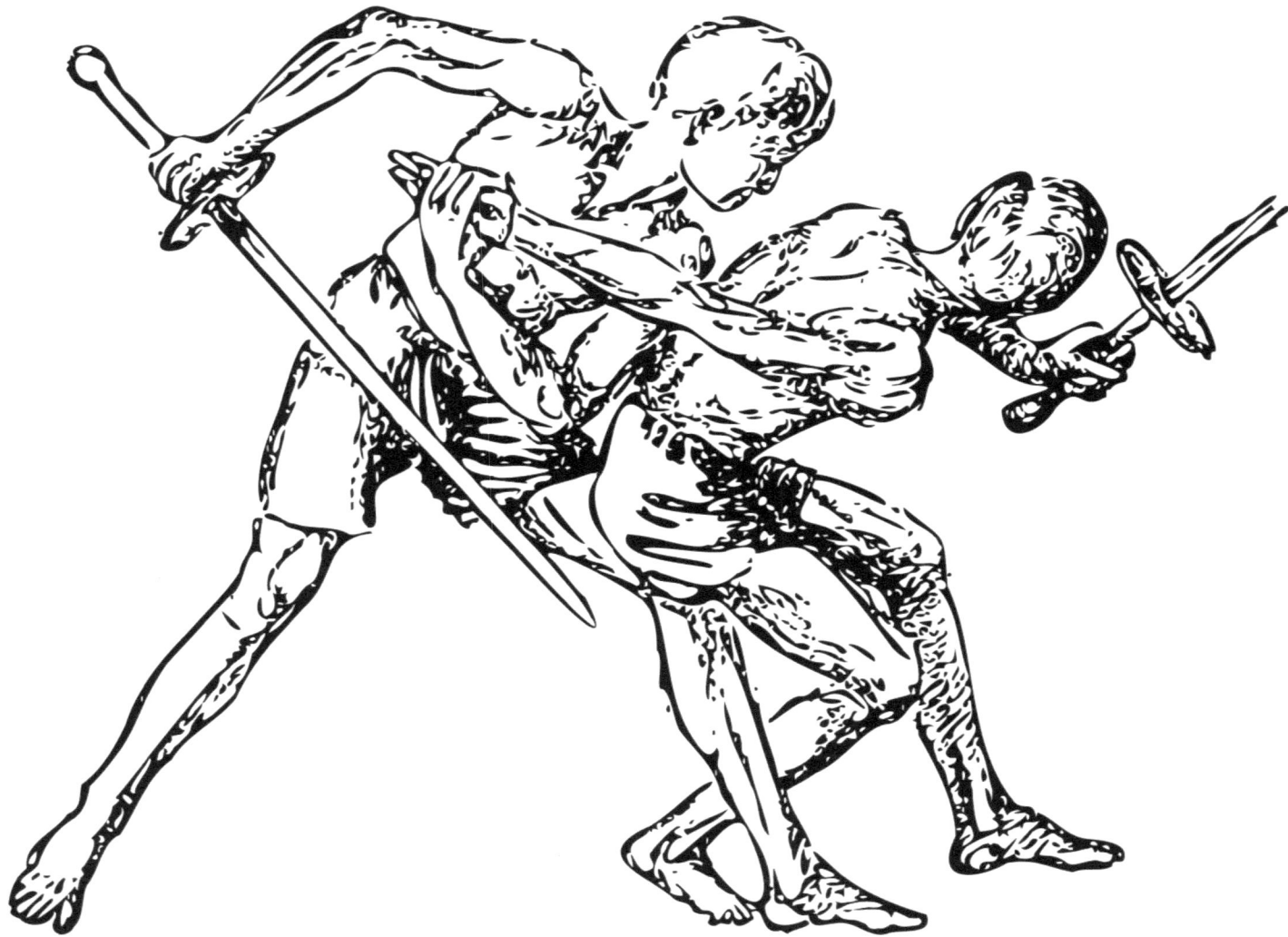

...and spin him quickly outwards and downwards. The adversary must spin himself and turn his back towards you. Then pull him over your forward leg—as is portrayed here—and so then he falls upon his back. That is also especially one right good greeting gesture for pleasant fellows.

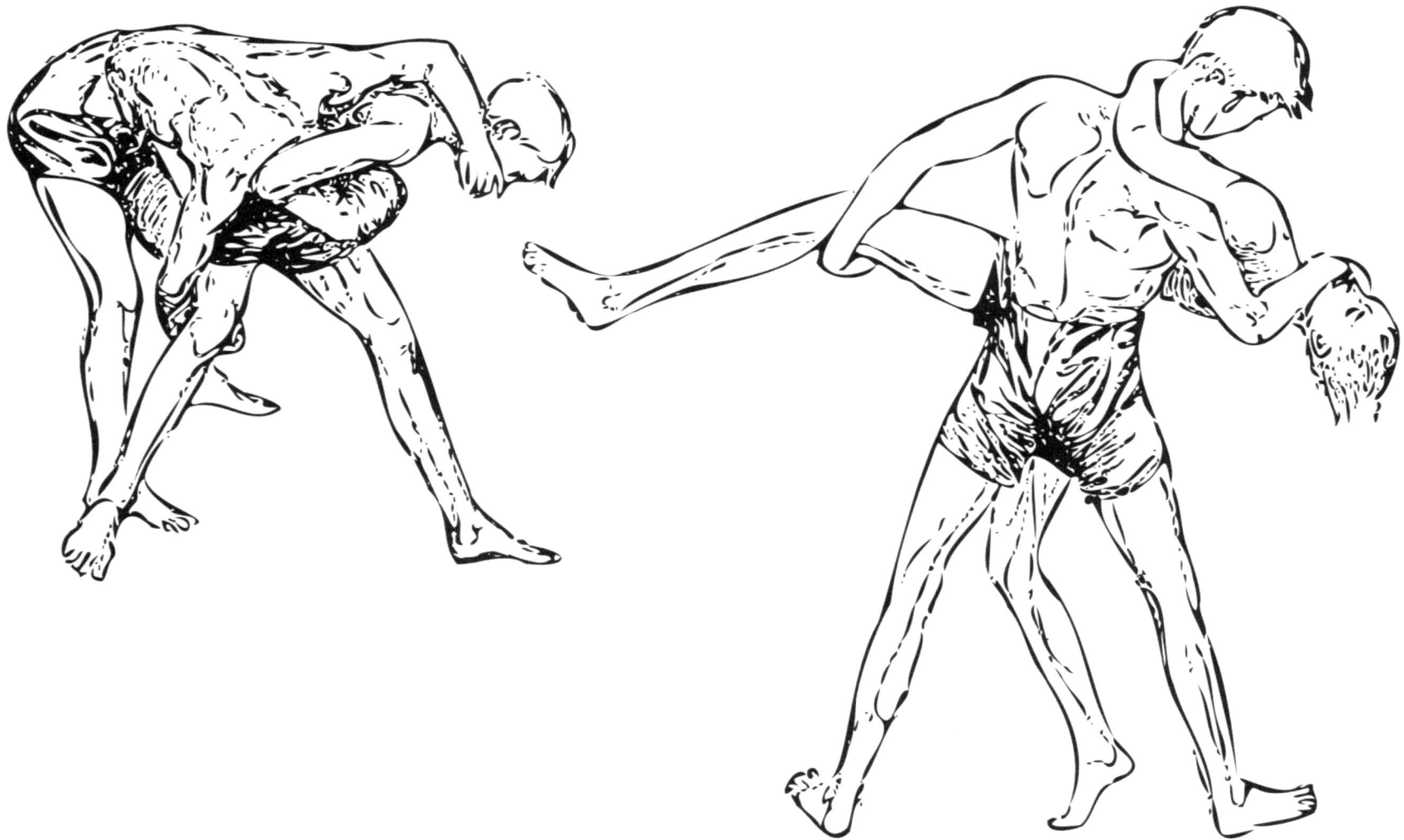

"Headlock" — The adversary has seized you around the neck, and he cannot throw you, so he would try to drag you out of the ring. So then with the one hand between your head and his head, seize him from behind and under his chin, while with the other hand into the knee-hollow—as portrayed here—press him backwards by his head and heave him high by one leg, thus he falls upon his back.

Closing

Swords high, as at the beginning, salute-hews towards both sides, swords to the left shoulders, handshake, about-turn, march off.

Outfit

The best fencing clothing are gym-shorts, because every hit and its nature are forthwith seen. However, it is regarded as a sign of good fencing when the hits are simultaneously energetic and light. That requires real domination of one's body, spirit, and weapon. Experientially, it is good or at least more pleasant, when the elbows are protected by leather cops and the ears by a rugby scrum-cap (and the eyes by sport-goggles).[18]

---

[18] Refer to the cheap, simple fencing outfit detailed in Rule 1 of the "Fencing Rules" later in this work.

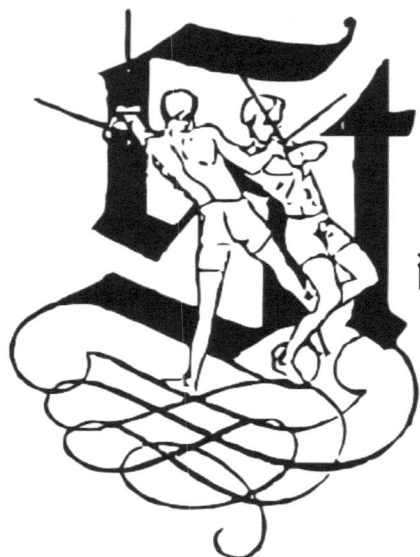

Stickfighting

Stickfighting is an exercise/training of courage, temper, flexibility, and decisiveness. The art of fencing with the stick poses similar demands as fencing with sabre and rapier: Correct timing, speed, and correct spacing.

"Timing" means acting decisively in the moment, when success promises.

"Speed" means, according to the composure of the adversary, swiftly deciding and executing the decision lightning-quick and definitively.

"Spacing" is the measure[19] from the adversary, in which you can hit the adversary, without exposing your own targets needlessly.

The main failures are: Stiffness, indecisive wavering or playing; fencing with the adversary's weapon instead of with the adversary himself; over-eagerness due to excitement, and lethargy due to laziness or cowardice; but then also straying from the dueling line and spoiling every clean bout through constant oblique cuts.

The (fencer's) power-expenditure should be as small as is still possible for victory. Only then is the fencing beautiful and artful.

Every hit should be as light as the nature of the weapon allows for it. That is chivalric/knightly as well as graceful. The entire fencing must make for an easy, safe, and clearly deliberate spectacle.

---

[19] Hull, *Mass.*

Foretraining

Some fundamental and ever-recurring movements and stances must be trained before beginning any further fencing bouts, such that they must be made correctly as a matter of course.

"Guard" means the composure wherefrom and whereout I can perform all cuts, diversions, and foot-motions easily and quickly, without offering the adversary even one inch more hit-area than is strictly needed. For hits as for diversions, I must dominate the fist-postures, with which the correct arm-motions automatically unite.

In order to gain the correct spacing and to keep the dueling line, all foot-motions must go automatically. In the bout there is no extra time for thinking. Pass, return to guard, stepping and springing both forward and backward, must be well-trained and must be exactly-gauged and controlled movements.

Any bout without the domination of hand, arm, and legs can only degenerate into foul play, whereby you kids never learn fencing, and which very soon makes for no more fun.

The Stick

This is simply a seasoned, perhaps finger-thick, ashen rod—although hazel and namely cherry or field-maple (hedge-maple) also work. It should be as straight as possible and somewhat flexible, otherwise it whips around every clean diversion and hits undeservingly.

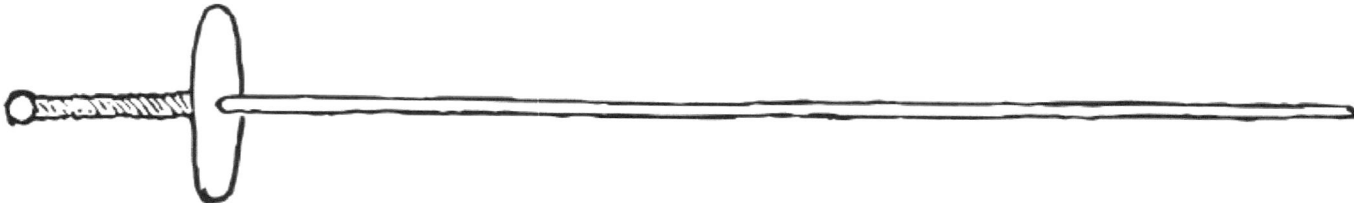

Length 108 cm, of which 18 cm are grip. For hand-guard a plywood disc or a sort of sabre-basket from steam-bent laminated wood (or simply wicker or leather) is needed. The "blade" is round, worked little or not, the grip is carved squarely. The hand-guard gets a corresponding four-cornered hole in the middle, and is shoved from below over the grip. This is then wrapped tightly and thickly with cord, such that the disc is set fast, and the hand grasps it comfortably.

The Dueling Line

This is a 10 meter-long straight line. At the beginning of a bout, the fencers form up along the dueling line, so that at basic stance, with outstretched arms and sticks, the stick-points contact each other over the middle of the dueling line. When the fencers stand correctly, the dueling line invariably passes through left heel and right foot of the one, and then through right foot and left heel of the other. It shall never be forsaken. Whoever forsakes it, despite warning, counts as hit.

Hand-Composures or Fist-Postures

1. Thumbnail downwards
2. Thumbnail leftwards
3. Thumbnail upwards
4. Thumbnail rightwards

The handgrips (shown on the following page) are intentionally roughly sketched. The stick shall always stay approximately in extension of the forearm, so that the cuts become hewn substantially from the forearm, not from the wrist. A convulsive clutching of the grip is then not possible.

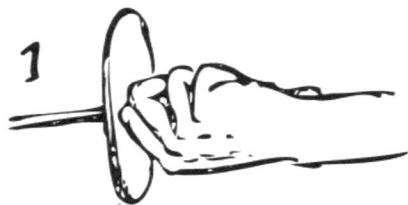

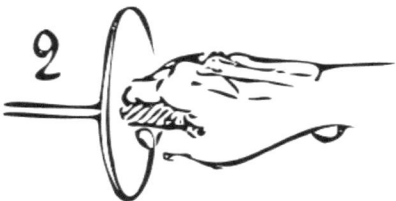

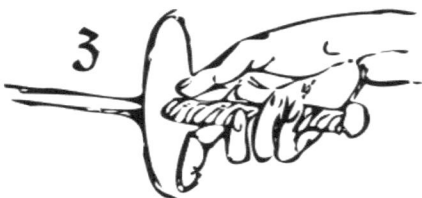

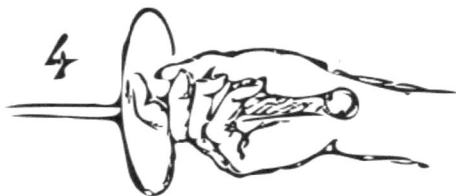

Basic Stance and Salute

Forming up along the dueling line, taking space, basic stance as illustrated.

For salute, a horizontal overhead twirling towards right and left is always stricken, then going into "guard."

For conclusion of the bout: From the last guard into the basic stance, twirling twice as at beginning, then basic stance, whereby the left hand supports the stick, then handshake with the adversary, about-turn, march off.

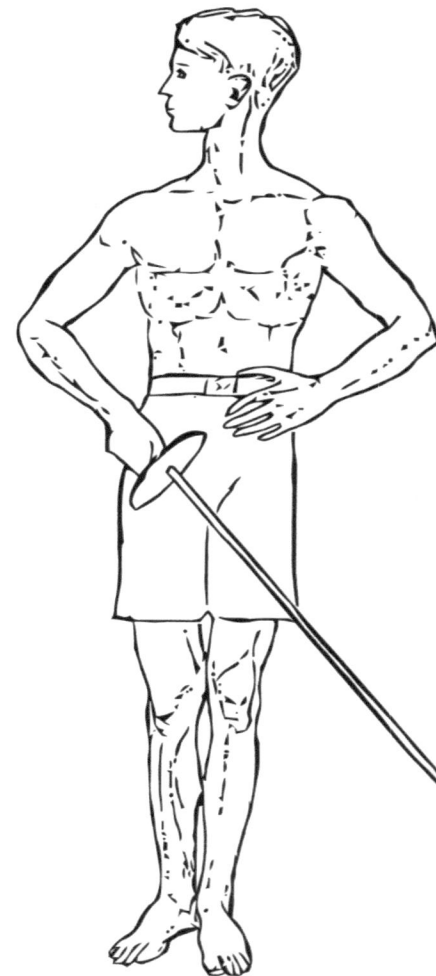

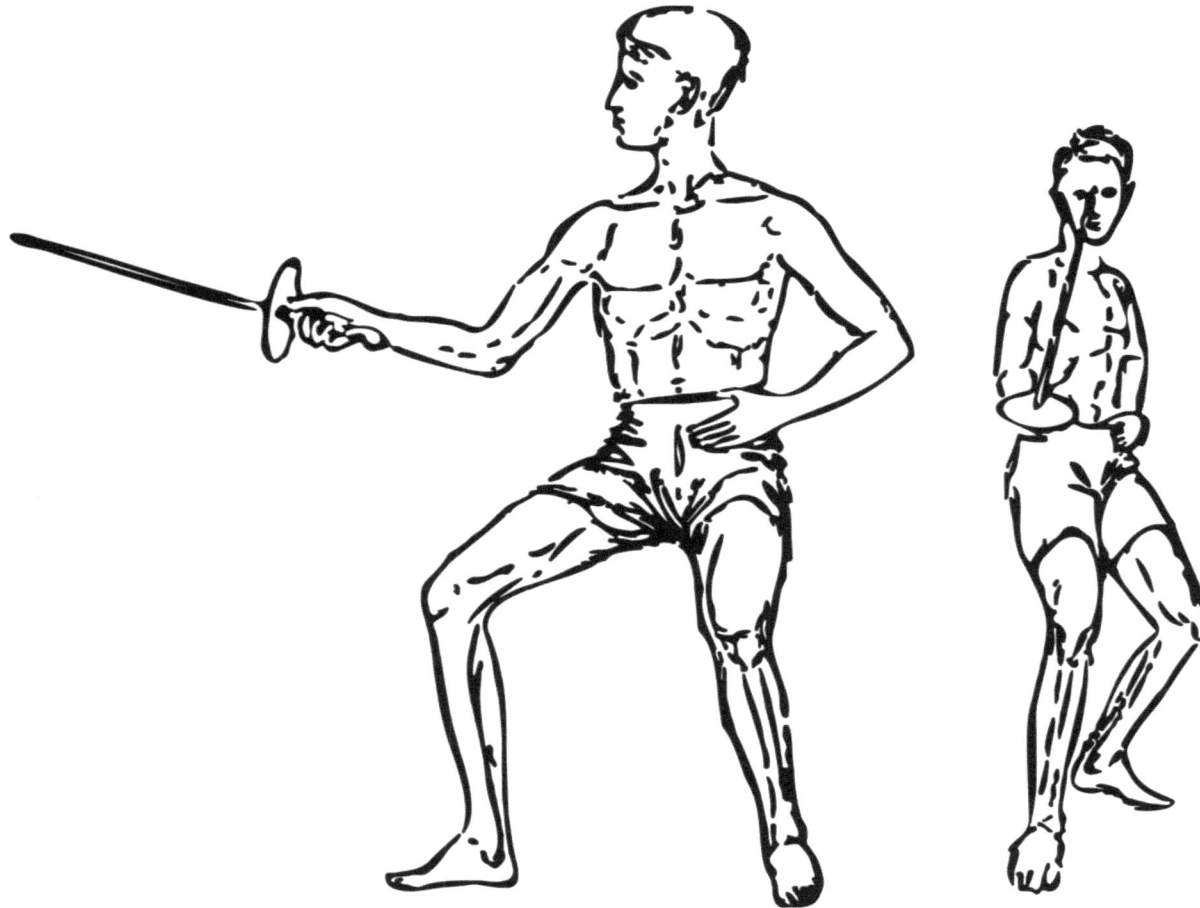

The Guard

This is the readiness stance. The most proper/likely is the third fist-posture as depicted previously. From here, I invite the adversary to an attack, while I expose my chest or my flank, then from there I attack with a lunge. Forearm and stick are roughly one straight punch, which aims at the brow of the adversary. The forearm must always stay behind the disc, in order not to become hit with an "arm-stop-cut." (Pull in the elbows!) The right foot is in directional alignment, the left foot perpendicular thereto. The feet have about two foot-lengths of spacing. The center-of-gravity is in the middle between both heels, always "squatting down" with elastic knees. The right leg never gets stretched, the left only by passing.

The Pass

This is the smallest possible attack-movement, which is needed, in order to reach the adversary. The hit must seat before the passing foot touches the floor, even when initially a feint is made. The supporting leg may slide neither from the floor nor away. The passing foot, by pass and return, must be solidly landed. This movement happens exactly in the directional alignment.

Foot-Motions

"Forward Step," exactly so far, such that the heel of the passing foot goes wherein the point of the foot was previously. The supporting leg accordingly goes after.

"Backward Step": The supporting leg treads back one foot-length, then the passing leg treads back.

"Forward Spring": Both feet—exactly in fencing stances and along the dueling line—make one flat spring forwards, only exactly so big as needed, and then you instantly attack!

"Backward Spring": The passing leg treads as far as possible behind the supporting leg—as depicted by the "arm-stop-cut"—which instantly follows into the corresponding stance.

Diversions

Head-cuts are forbidden, thusly abolished at least ideally, because welts across the face are not really pretty, yet (fencers) are the more hearty for it. Therewith also abolished are the corresponding diversions, the first, fifth and sixth of sabre fencing lore. In an emergency, if a cut upon the chest or arm goes somewhat high, the third and fourth diversions must be deployed accordingly high.

While stickfighting, the diverting motion cannot be entirely precisely executed because of the incidental pliability of the weapon; rather it must be somewhat nearer to the body yet broader, such that the stick of the adversary does not hit by whipping around.

The Cuts

These are not hard strikes, rather short sharp slashes. There "upon the blank pelt" is it fought, where any hit is to be seen as a small red stripe. It is a sign of good fencing, when these stripes are entirely short and fine. When hostile cuts fall, causing welts upon the adversary, these could result in such a cut released upon the chest of the hostile fencer, which this "hacker" may not divert.

There are the following cuts:
Chest-Cut, Belly-Cut (20 cm lower than chest), those are the cuts upon the inside of the right-handed fencer.

Cuts upon the right flank and the right forearm are the cuts upon the outside of the right-handed fencer. Outside there are a whole bunch of special cuts with the selfsame hit-aiming which are beyond acknowledgement of the illustrations and their text. There are to be no thrusts.

Hit-areas go from neck until waist inclusively, or until the upper border of the fencer's gym-shorts or swim-trunks.

Feints or sham-cuts, equally sham-cuts and countercuts:
All feints must clearly distinguish themselves from senseless gesticulating, whereby they become cleanly "withdrawn" ("withdrawing" = backswing) and, like real cuts, actually threaten the adversary. They shall mislead the adversary to diverting motions towards one side, so that a speedy cut can land upon the other side.

Feints and cuts must be performed in a single pass. There are not to be cuts upon the face and the head; nor also are any feints to be made towards their direction.

Double-Feints (e.g. chest-feint—flank-feint—belly-cut) can still be valid, but only so, when they become performed very quickly and precisely. The fencer, who deploys double-feints, must manage two feints and one cut during a single pass, because otherwise he gives the adversary the right to an interim cut during the then-delayed attack.

Such "cuts in the tempo" mostly hit, are in reality only just delayed attacks allowed in, and only have validity as hits when the performing fencer does not become hit thereby. Cuts upon the opposing weapon so to strike it out the hand, and upon the hand so to make it numb, are not to be done. Whereas so-called "glide-cuts" can still be hewn, by which one's own weapon glides along the opposing weapon, forces it off the line, so then to hit into the target.

Widely-extended diversions can also be validly swept out by the return motion, thus as it were, with the back edge.

The countercuts are especially vital, because after diverting an attack, then from that diversion those immediately threaten the possibly-not-yet-again-ready adversary. It is therefore equally vital, not to put an attack further forward, as it is tolerable for one's own safety before the adversary's countercut, and forthwith to counterhew open up any diversion.

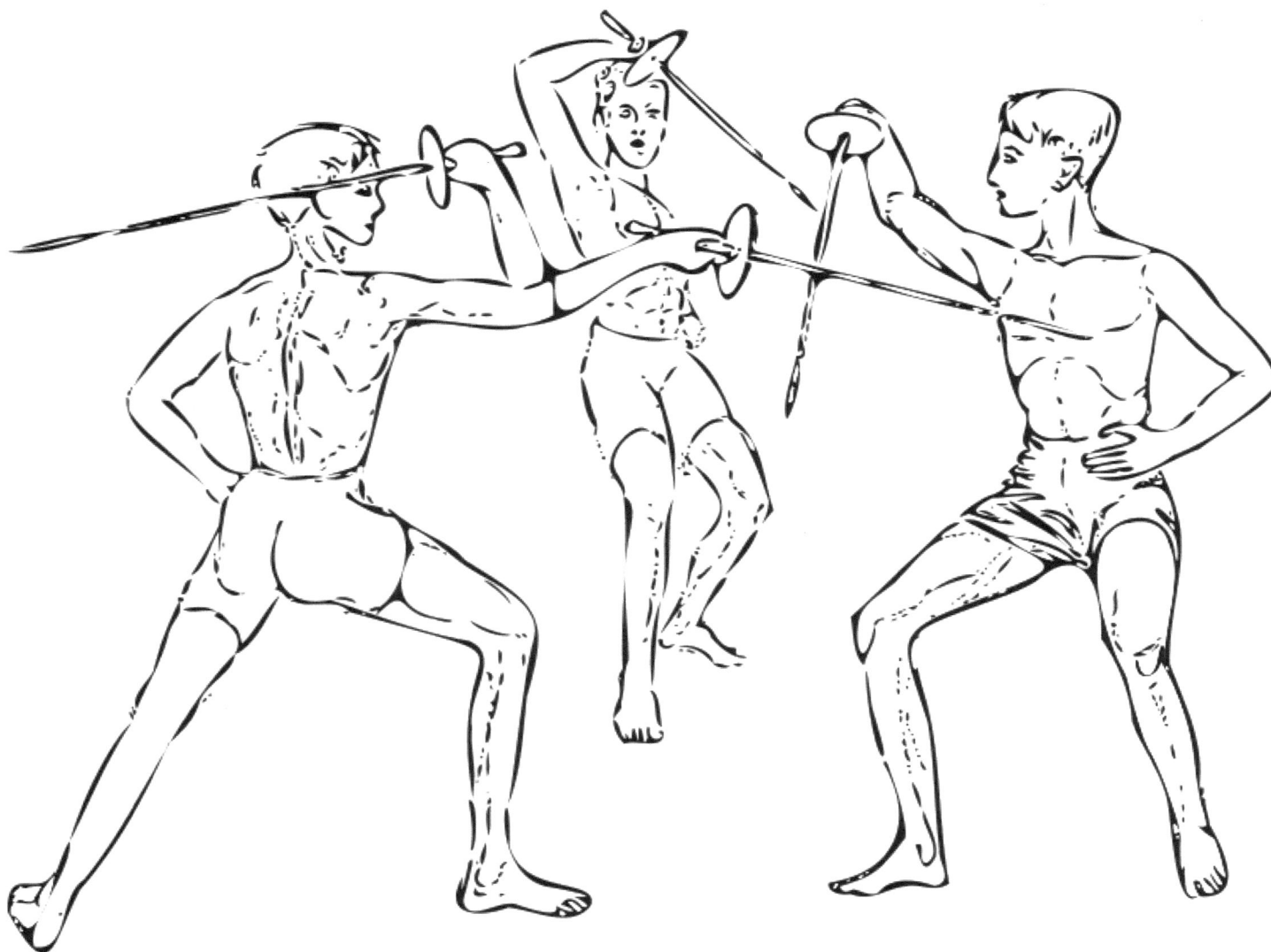

A high chest-cut by the left fencer is held off in the first diversion by the right fencer. From here, either a chest-cut or a quick cut towards the right flank of the adversary can become counterhewn. (The third illustrated fencer simply shows, from the front, how he does warding with the first diversion.)

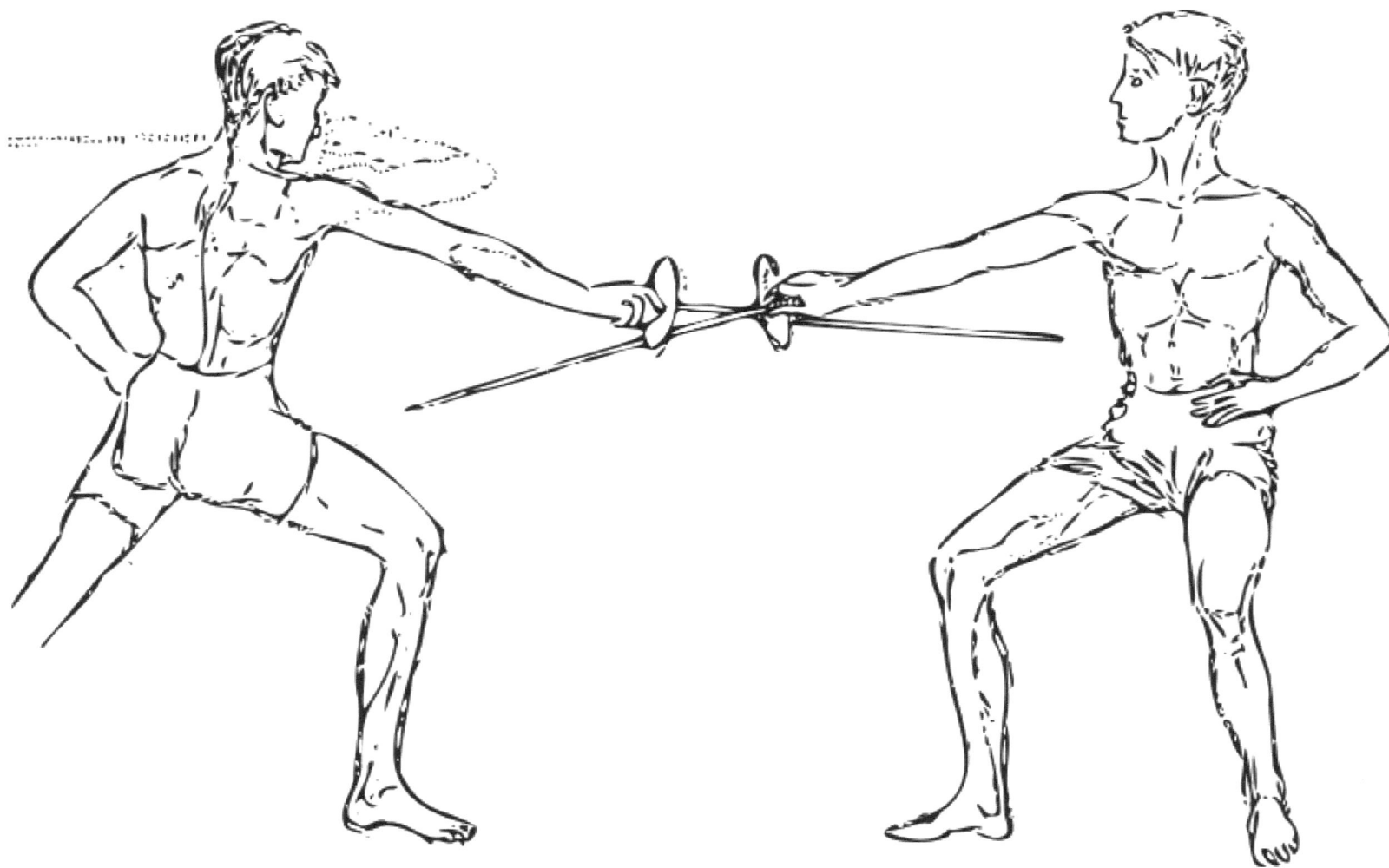

The left fencer strikes a flanking cut. The right fencer is in the second diversion. From here, the fencing arm becomes somewhat withdrawn perpendicular to the countercut, and then chest or flank becomes hewn; or one deep belly-cut during the return motion from the diversion, provided this were put far enough forward.

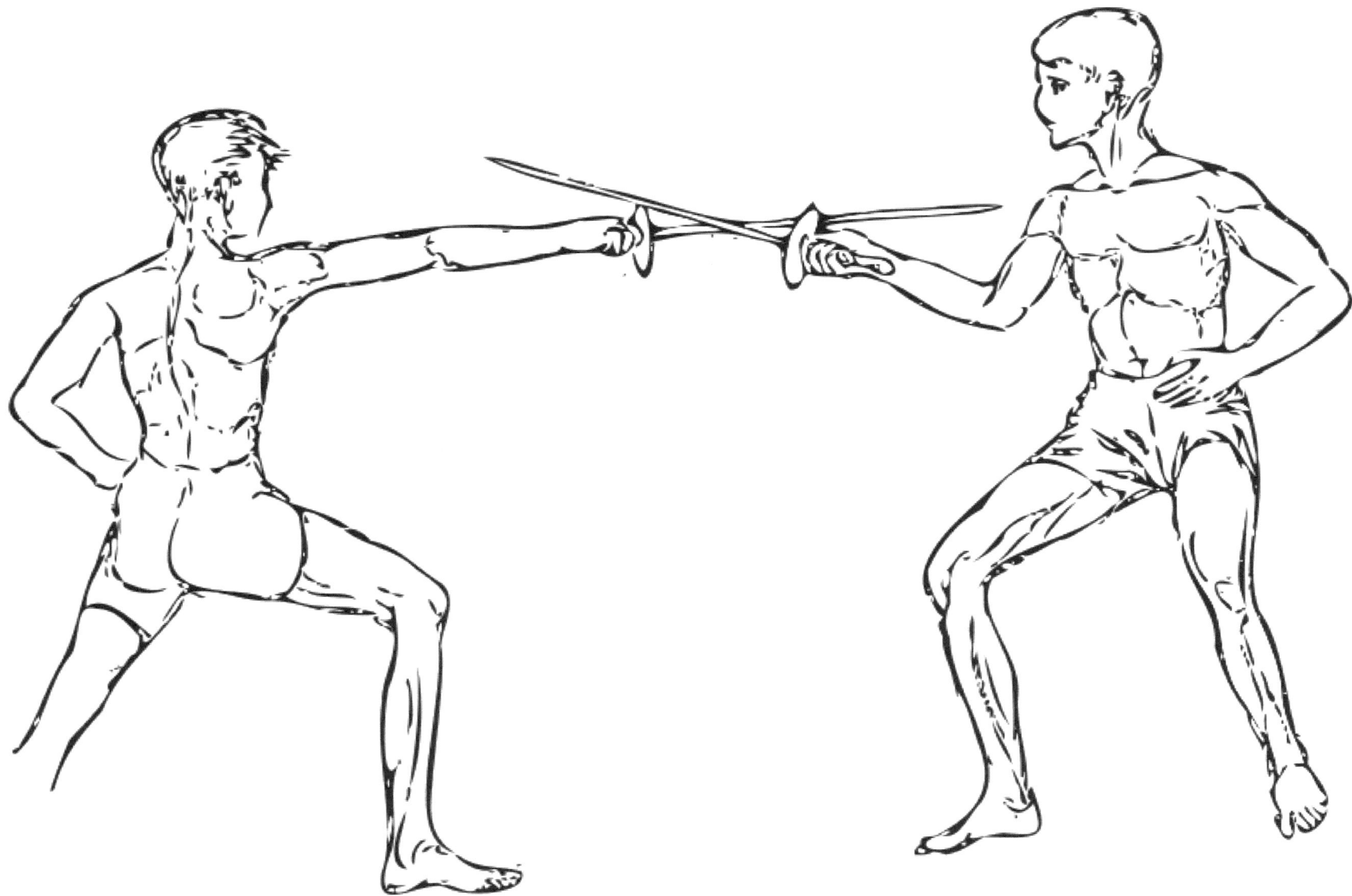

High flanking cut (forearm-cut) diverted in third diversion. The best counterstrike is to low flank.

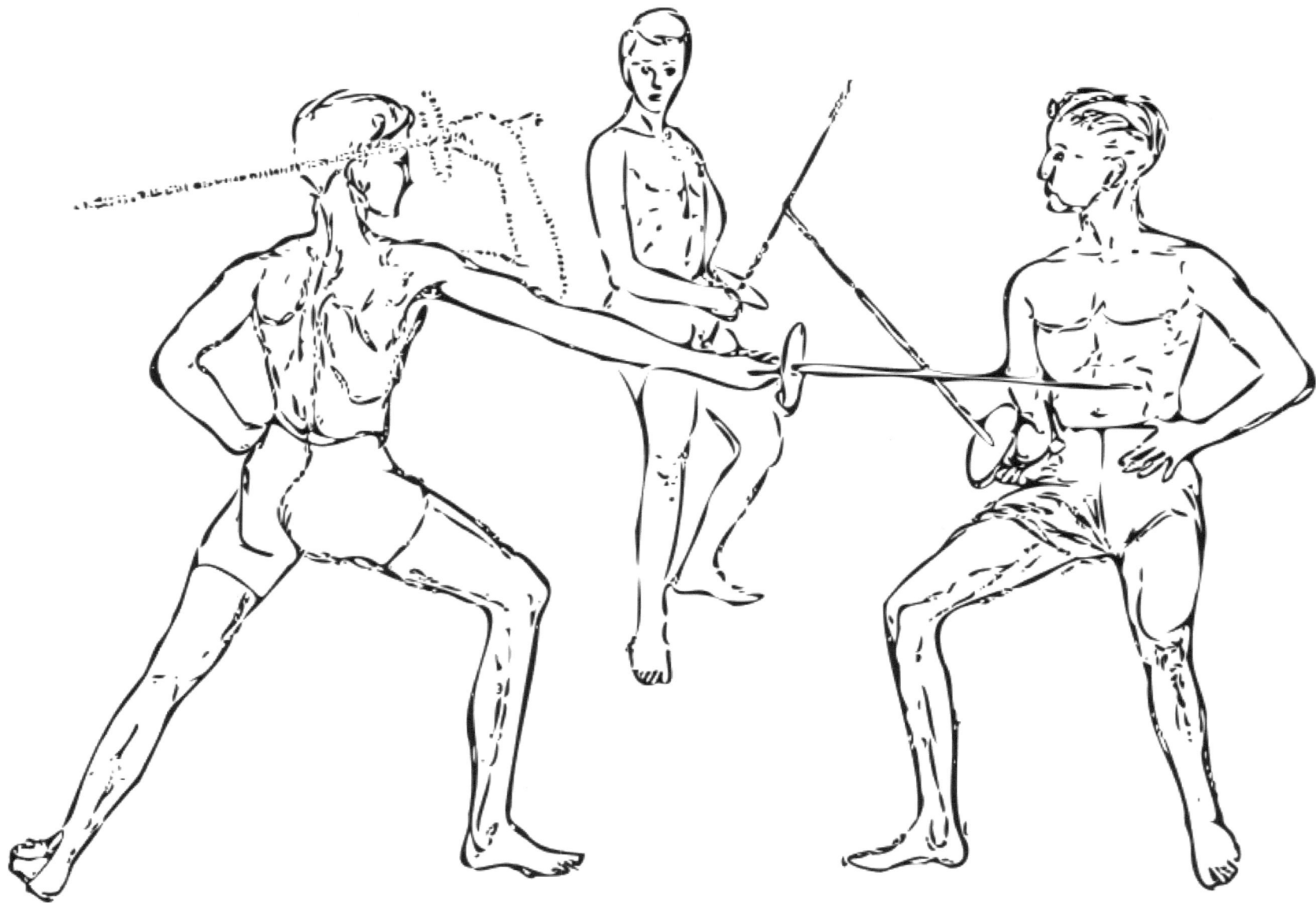

Belly-cut diverted in fourth diversion. Best countercut is again belly-cut or chest-cut. The third fencer shows, from the front, the fourth diversion.

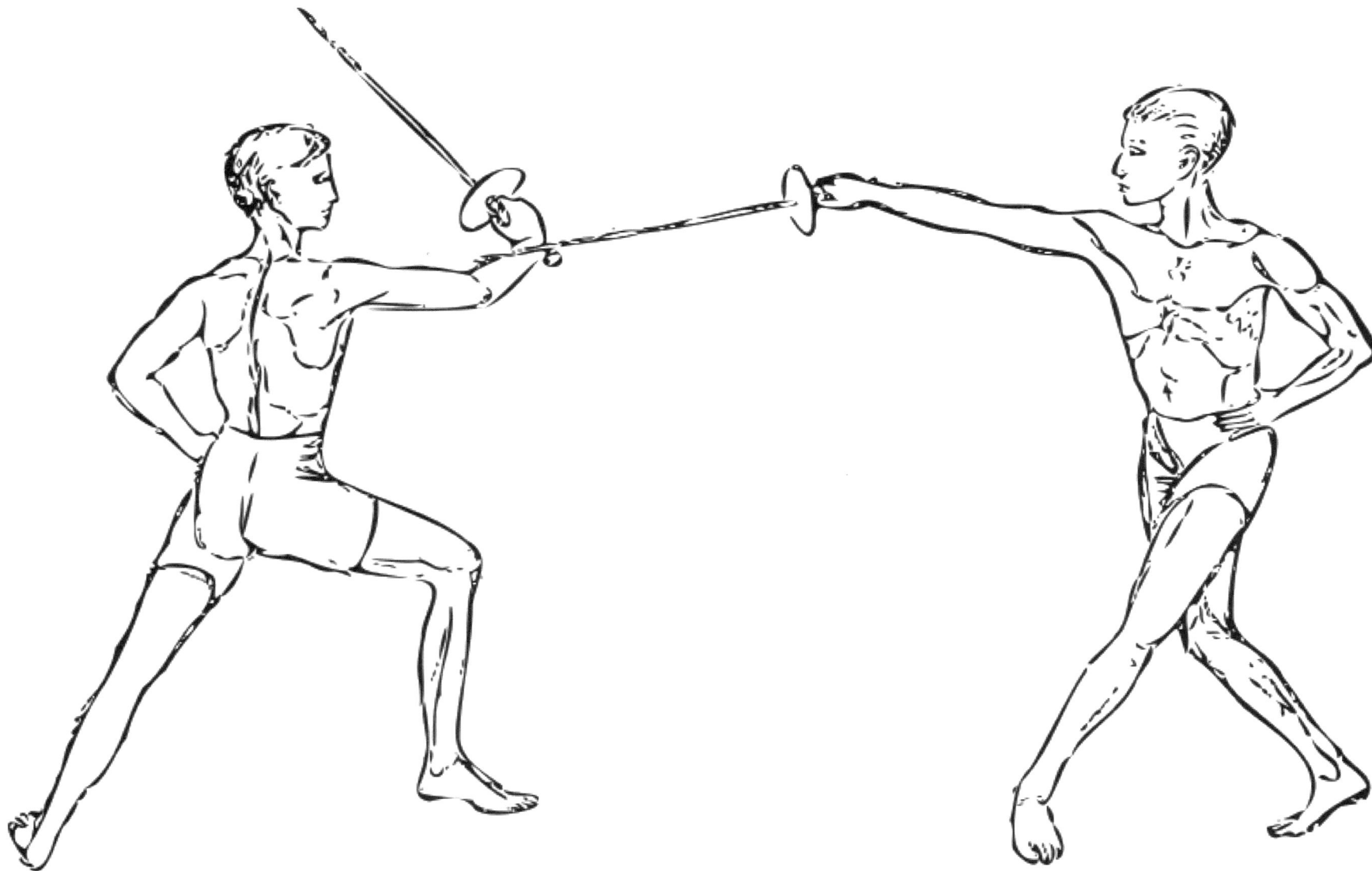

The left adversary is on the attack. The right fencer hits while retreating—by springing backwards—with an arm-stop-cut to the forearm of the attacker. This cut only has validity—like all attacking cuts—when oneself does not get hit thereby. It is only possible when the adversary is too slow, and thereby he so exposes his forearm, as shown here.

Left-Handed Fencers

Firstly, all these rules are valid for right-handed fencers: Against left-handed fencers the cuts and the fist-postures remain the same, however e.g. a flanking cut hits the belly of a left-handed fencer, a chest-cut hits his fencing arm, etc. The guard of the left-handed fencer is naturally inverted from that of the right-handed fencer, thus his outside is the left, his inside is the right.

Bout-Training

Until the fencers dominate the aforesaid movements, stances, diversions, and cuts, then they shall fence according to command. Thus the sports-teacher orders e.g. 1. Attack with chest-cut; 2. Divert with fourth diversion and strike at flank (or simply) 2. Strike at flank. Then 1. Go into second diversion, and during the return motion to guard, strike with belly-cut; 2. Divert with the fourth diversion and strike flank again. This proceeds until *Halt!* is called.

That then is trained—naturally always while switching roles—until all is performed cleanly. In order not to fumble, every fencer allows an undiverted cut here and there, which then must doubtlessly hit. (Otherwise, the adversary has fought to the stick instead of to the man. He must therefore take a free cut to his chest!)

When the free bouting begins, at least one judge must stand on each side, for correcting mistakes and deciding hits. Because every hit is to be seen, then but little doubt can emerge.

"Thrashing" easily makes one better. By brawling with the single stick, there goes not only the defunct but also the artistic of all fencing. It is the best method for never learning clean fencing. Because our youth, as widely acknowledged, have ice-water flowing through their veins, frivolity with the sticks must indeed be prevented, for that is always the prelude to any better thrashing.[20]

Dueling

Brawlers, big-talkers, and braggarts get the chance to present proof, by stickfighting with the adversary, that the correct relationship still survives between champ and chump. Instead of quarreling for hours and finally scrapping formlessly, let the adversaries compete against each other, with single sticks and without shirts, to show who is better at the vital qualities of composure and temper. Weeping is quite disallowed, but is no scandal, when fencing continues cleanly nonetheless. However, the director is therefore equally responsible for discontinuing any rudeness and any ridiculous demands by young scamps.[21] The youth should hammer, not tap, each other. Stage short bouts with a previously-agreed hit-score. A bout to 5 at most 10 hits is perfectly sufficient. There is not to be bouting until fatigue. No bout shall last longer than 10 to 15 minutes maximum. Fencing training is not to be longer than 30 minutes.

Fencing Rules

1. The competitive duels happen outdoors in front of the squad to which the fencers belong. Outfit: Shorts (plus cup) and sneakers. Work/Tactical-goggles or motorcycle-goggles are proper. It is sufficient to wear a thick rugby scrum-cap or trusty hockey-helmet.[22] For trained fencers, no protection is needed.

---

[20] German idioms and irony run rampant throughout here, hence my contextual rendering.
[21] Scamps (Pimpfe) was a Scouting term of fond mockery for the youngest boys of the German Youngfolk (Deutsches Jungvolk).
[22] Viable/Additional modern safety equivalents contextually translated by me for benefit of modern reader/fencer.

2. The combatants subject themselves to the fencing rules and without contradicting the dueling judge.

3. The fencers are marshalled via challenging, whereupon it is just self-evidently honorable to challenge a strong and dangerous adversary.

4. Hit-areas are torso and fencing arm from neck until belt, including or until the upper border of the swim-trunks or gym-shorts.

5. The dueling judge draws the dueling line and makes sure, by distancing them, that the stick-points contact each other precisely over its middle. Then stances are taken by the combatants. The bout begins at the command of *Go!* The dueling judge prevents any premature attack.

6. When there is a hit then the judge, who first notices it, orders *Halt!* Then the adversaries go into basic stances. Resumption of the bout from the middle, as stated above.

7. Synchronous hits by both sides each count, if both fencers were on the attack; otherwise the attacker gains the advantage.

8. If any bout degenerates into roughhousing, it gets broken up by the dueling referee. The fencers are then admonished. If only one fencer is guilty, the other fencer gains one free cut which the guilty may not divert (yet may dodge). It becomes counted, but not used, so as to take revenge.

9. When an adversary loses his stick, the other adversary chivalrously uplifts and freezes his own. Hits upon the unarmed adversary—also when he shatters his stick—are invalid; unless it can be supposed that the stick has been thrown away; which the dueling judge ultimately decides.

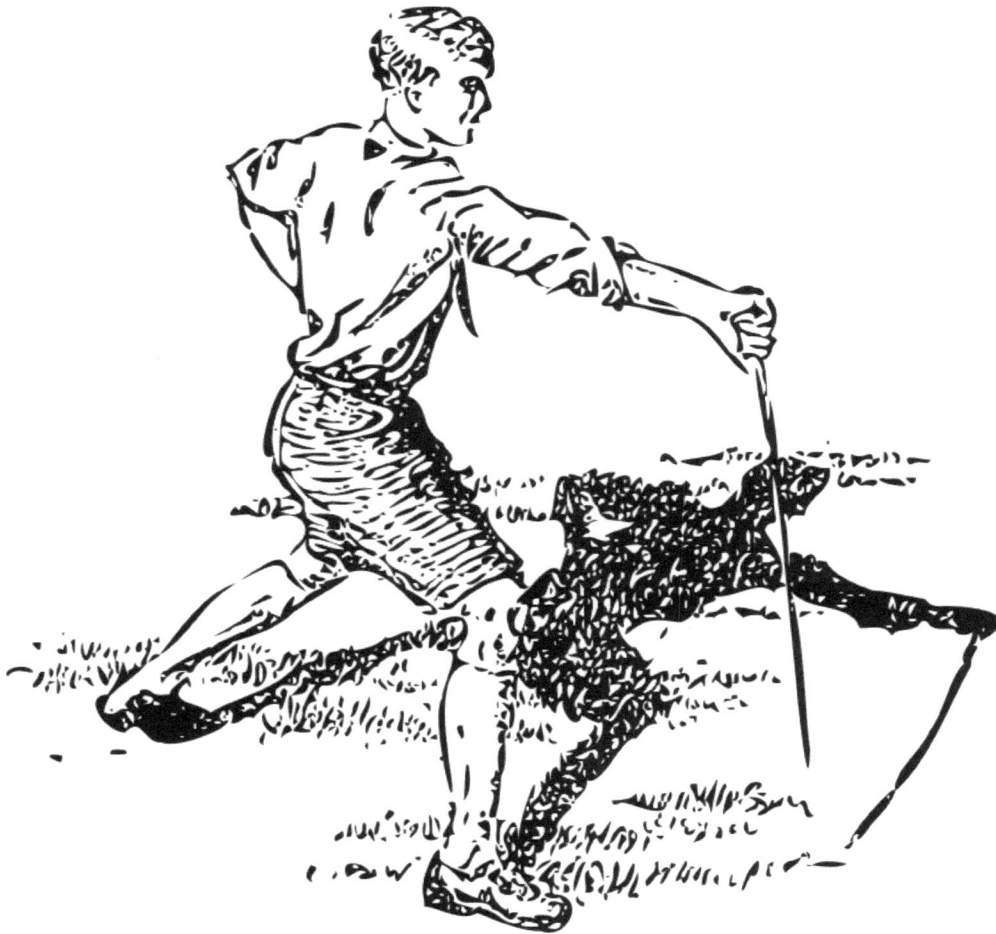

10. Except for when asked by the dueling judge, the combatants are forbidden to speak even during the combat-breaks, which are needed for verification of hits. Malcontention leads to terminating the bout forthwith and sending the guilty one away. After completion, every bout is to be reviewed.

11. The duration of any bout shall not exceed 15 minutes. After 3 hits or 7 minutes, sides are switched. So then the fencers go past one another, left-to-left, with their sticks upraised. Each one takes the position previously held by his adversary.

12. Both the umpires or dueling judges—even better four!—convey their observations to the dueling referee. Then this referee decides the fight conclusively and uncontestably.

FINISHED! GO!

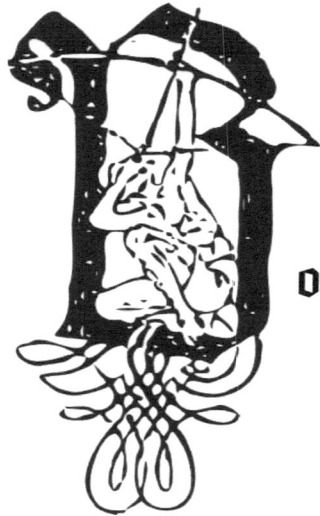

Bowshooting / Archery

The bow, even today, is the silent weapon-of-need for the last primitive human tribes, e.g. upon Sakhalin and Formosa, upon Malaita and Madagascar, in Annam and Tonquin. Their quality and potency are acknowledged by the fact that the French bringers of Christian culture advance against them with gas-grenades.[23]

For us, the bow is also more than a pretty toy: a sporting weapon that demands prowess, body-control, and shooter-education to master.

Shooting proficiency can be achieved with a well-shapen bow and with well-feathered and cleanly-carven arrows, whereupon you become astounded at yourself as soon as you have done some training. I have seen Youngfolk scamps shooting 8 to 10 of a dozen arrows into a 40 cm target at 40 paces range, and 12- to 14-year-old youth shooting a good-far 150 meters with a light sporting bow.

There are good and capable bows for purchase everywhere, which are a composite of two woods. However, they require very good treatment, especially of the bowstring,[24] and almost always break when the bowstring misfortunately snaps or when they are wrongly strung. So we must shoot—at least until we can command and handle this weapon generally—just homemade cheap bows.

The bow must absolutely have the following properties: It must be adapted/matched to the height and strength and size and prowess of the shooter. Notably, when he may not happen to be too strong.

---

[23] These statements were all quite correct circa 1935.
[24] *Sehne* was an original term which can mean both "bowstring" and "sinew."

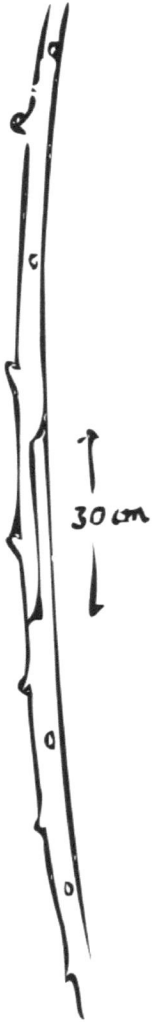

It must have consistent propulsion / quickening. Thus it must not be made of green wood nor become wet. It must not flake nor indeed rend apart from ordinary strain. It must—at least for us—be cheap. So first we build ourselves a simple bow. The best kinds of wood are:

Yew *(taxus baccata)*: Since there is not any yew wood which be twig/knot-free plus correspondingly long and strong,[25] then a yew bow always looks rough. Regarding any little twigs, 2 cm long twig-stubs must stay in place, lest the bow break at some cut-off site. If needed, the bow can be fashioned of two limbs that are glued and bound together at the middle (as illustrated).

Elm: Elm bows are very capable. The field-elm (white elm) is better than the mountain elm.

Maple: The best is the field-maple (hedge-maple). The bow shall be so long that it goes from fingertips to fingertips with your arms outstretched sideways.[26]

The middle part of the bow—about 30 cm—is left round and shall itself not actually bow/bend.

Also, across the whole outside/face of the bow, its finest wood-grain must not be gashed. It is best to leave the bark on the wood until it falls off by itself via drying. In any event, it must not be peeled off with a knife nor knocked off! Likewise, entirely shaping the wood of the inside/back must be done. Before it is finished, file (do not cut!) the nocks for the bowstring into the bow-tips; then tiller the bow with cordage, so as to see whether the bow bends evenly.

---

[25] Much yew wood, even from the trunk, is knotty and twisted, thus unsuitable for bowmaking.
[26] Also the traditionally recommended length for an ashen quarter staff.

The shaping is done first with the knife, then with the rasp, file, and sandpaper. Finally, all the wood gets well-lacquered, because it warps if it absorbs moisture.

If the bow must be constructed of two pieces, then it is important that the overlapping limbs get very evenly matched, well-glued, and tightly wrapped. The wrapping is also glued, then lacquered. Any cracked or chipped lacquer anywhere must be recoated forthwith.

As soon as small splinters spring up anywhere on the bow, or it frays, that site must get well-wrapped (twine and glue). Then it holds again perfectly. Without this care, it breaks up shallow or deep at such a site.

If the bow is not used for a while then the bowstring is to be taken off and the bow hung up by its top end.

The Arrow or Shaft

Even a middling bow lets you shoot tolerably well, but only when the arrows are good! With bad arrows, even the best shooter with the best bow can hit nothing. Foremost, the arrows must be totally straight, otherwise they have already swerved while slipping from the bow.

The arrows must all be the same weight, because otherwise a special aiming point must be tried for each individual arrow.

The arrows must be correctly and exactly fletched; either so that they soar, as it were, without spinning; or so that they rotate exactly around the longitudinal axis; but in any event not wobbling. The arrows must always be completely smooth and clean.

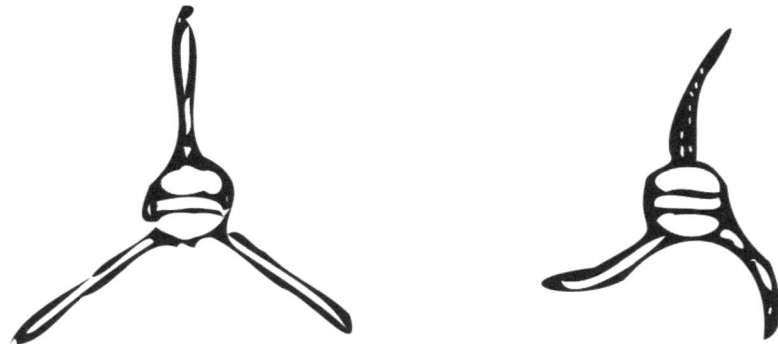

Every bit of clinging dirt reduces hit-scores.

From good air-dried ash wood or—when it shall be easier to carve and cheaper—from spruce wood, let the carpenter saw totally straight, twig/knot-free staves, about 60 cm long. Arrows must then be very carefully carved round, filed, and polished, until they are about pencil-thick (8 mm). Ash arrows shall then weigh about 25 g each, spruce arrows accordingly less, but in any event, all of them of exactly the same kind of wood. Then the notch is filed in precisely across the growth-rings. (Not cut!)

Then look as you let the arrow turn upon its point, and if it still seems to be a little crooked, then bend it straight over the campfire. So you can also produce very simple and cheap arrows from rods of dried hazel or dogwood (whipple), but from deep/sharp shots they easily fracture. Turkey or bustard feathers are best suited for fletching. The feathers of farm geese and all chickens are not suitable. Greylag goose feathers are better.

All three feathers of an arrow must be from the same wing! A vane is stripped off the quill, well-soaked in water, and glued onto the arrow with the bottom end against and exactly perpendicular to the nock. This is the "index feather."

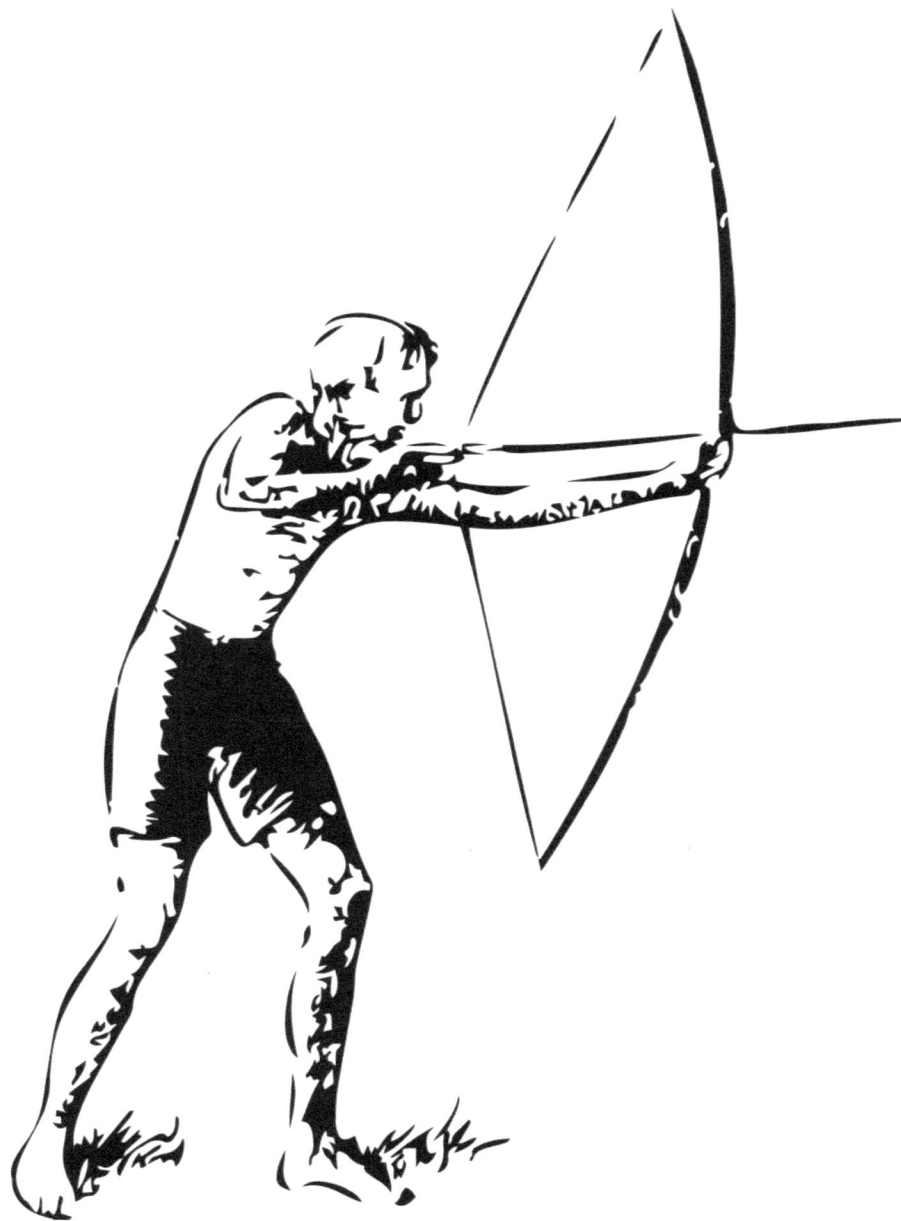

Then two more feather-vanes are made ready and glued so that they each juxtapose below the index feather at the same angle and at equal distance. The feathers, when they sit well and precisely, are tightly wrapped with fine thread and lacquered. The index feather is colorfully inked or painted. Also, you can file the arrow-points out of steel plate yourself; then cement and tightly wrap those into notches filed into and across the growth-rings at the top ends of the arrows. Well-proven have been old spitzer/spire bullets,[27] from which the leaden cores are smelted out; or also the slender points from worn-out dame-style umbrellas.

The bowstring must be very carefully crafted. It must neither stretch nor shrink in wet weather, nor snap without warning. Ordinary twine, kite-string, or fishing line just do not work. The best is 5- thread-thick "shoemaker-cord," well-waxed against wetness, and fortified at the ends by thickening with about 5 more threads. The bowstring is then spun out of three such strands, which must always project about one span beyond the ends of the bow. (30 cm longer than the bow.) Naturally, fortifying the ends must not emerge suddenly, rather it must merge gradually with the standard thickness.

A loop is spliced at one end of the finished, fortified, and triple-spun bowstring. This loop of the bowstring is slipped over the bottom end of the bow. The other end of the bowstring is slipped around the bow, by one handwidth just under its top horn, with a timber hitch—as illustrated. Now the bow—only as illustrated!—can become strung.

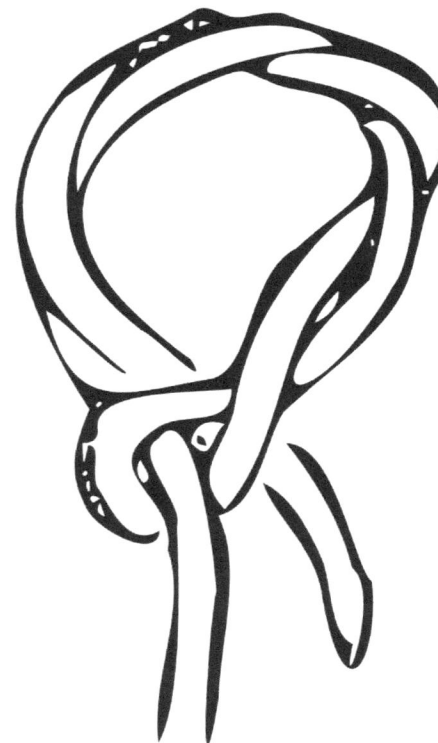

---

[27] S-Geschosse = Spitzgeschosse (pointed bullets): There were many of these small grim artifacts from the First World War to be found circa 1935, which were spent military bullets having copper/steel jackets and tips, and once hollowed by lead-removal, made suitable field-points for mounting onto arrow-shafts.

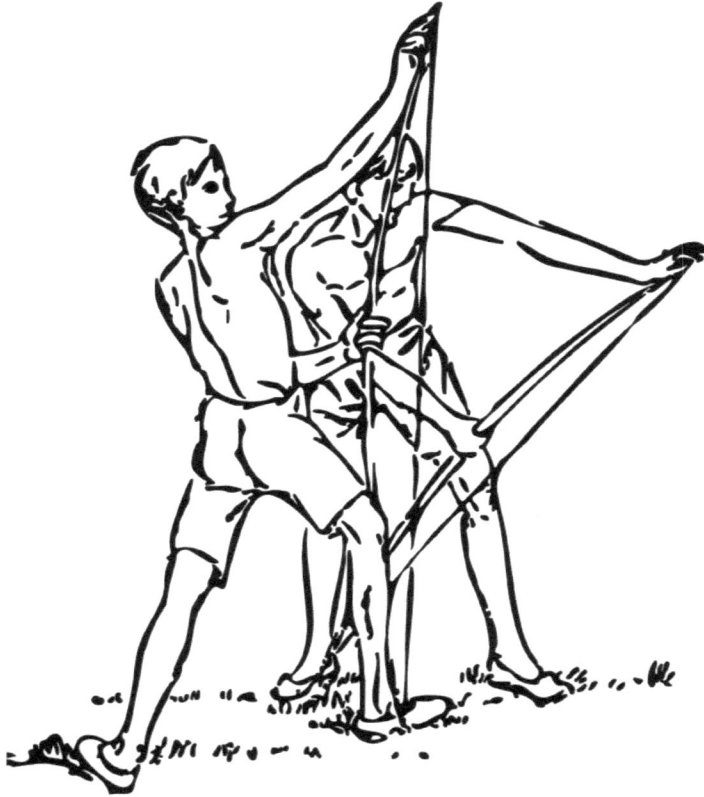

"Stringing" means spanning the bowstring over both ends of the bow, thusly tensed so its middle is spaced about 1/10 of its own length from the bow-arch.

Apart from the already-reinforced ends, the bowstring gets especially strained at its middle, where the arrow-nock rubs it. Thus here it must get a protective wrapping. So that it does not go loose, it must be done correctly, as illustrated.

Shooting Range and Targets

Since archery is not completely hazard-free, then it must be managed, so that there is the least possible chance for misfortune to befall. This is why you had best shoot across an old 50-meter small-caliber rifle-shooting range. Almost as good, and better suited to the nature of the weapon, is a straight forest lane / firebreak. When needed, either a clay quarry or a meadow swathe also works.

The shooting field must, firstly, prevent any danger for all invited and uninvited guests and spectators; and secondly, warrant that not only poorly shot but also untimely runaway arrows are found again. Thirdly, there shall be neither stones nor iron parts whereupon the arrows could split / shatter.

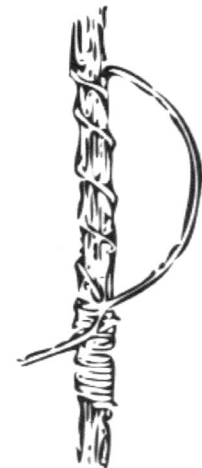

The target shall equal so many centimeters diameter as the paces away that you are shooting. A colorful cardboard disc against a turf-wall/haystack suffices. This can also be artfully replicated by stuffing pieces of turf/sod into a large flat packing box. When placed, it gets slanted facing somewhat skywards, so that the arrows hit and stick at about right angles. Sandbags also work, when the sand is not hard-packed, as well as wet clay.

Shooting Instructions

Standing and Gripping: With rifle and crossbow, the shooter shoots directly through it; yet with the bow, the shooter shoots from just beside it. A line drawn through both your aligned heels must aim at the target. The left archer of the illustration is correct, the right archer is wrong.

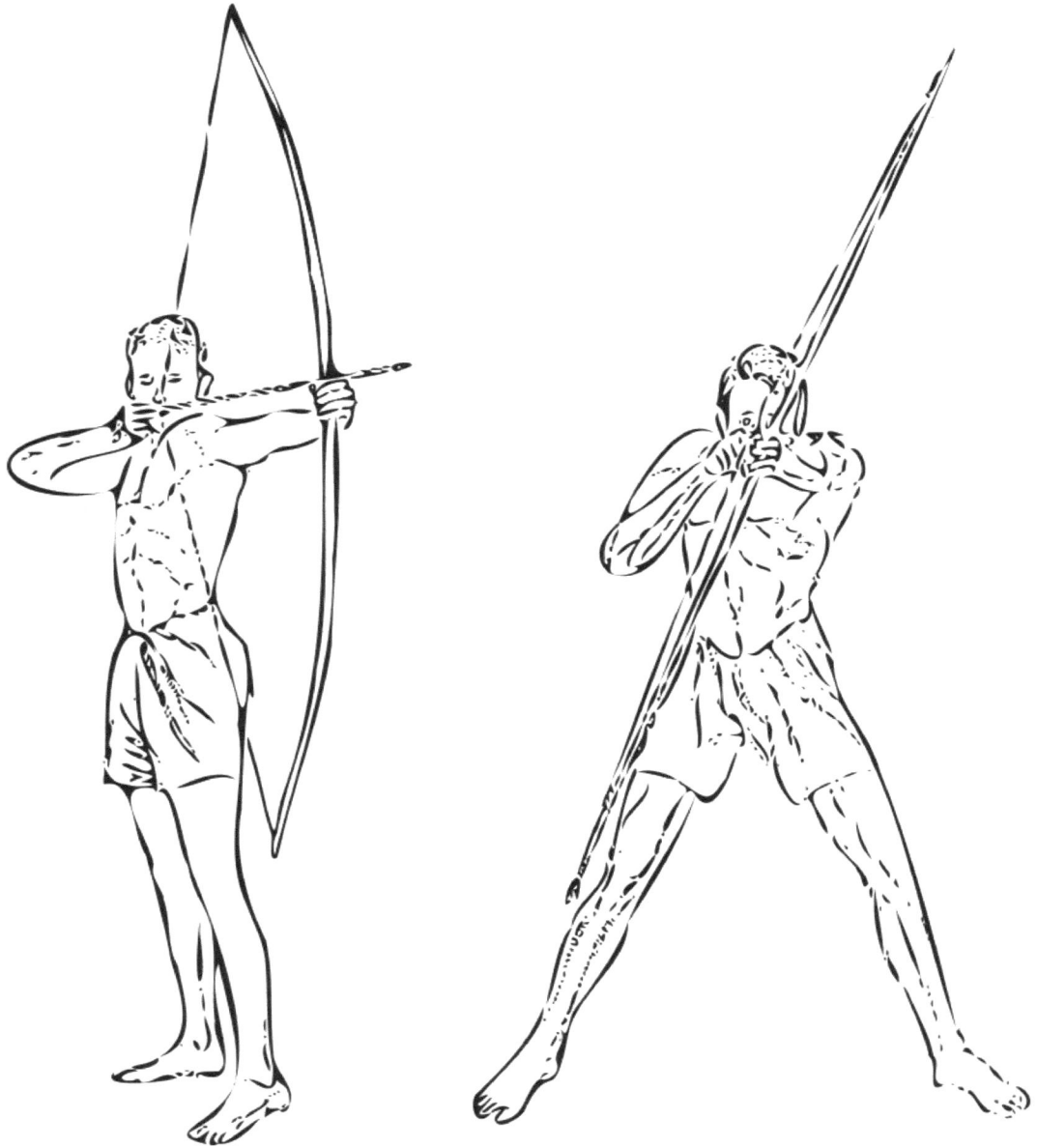

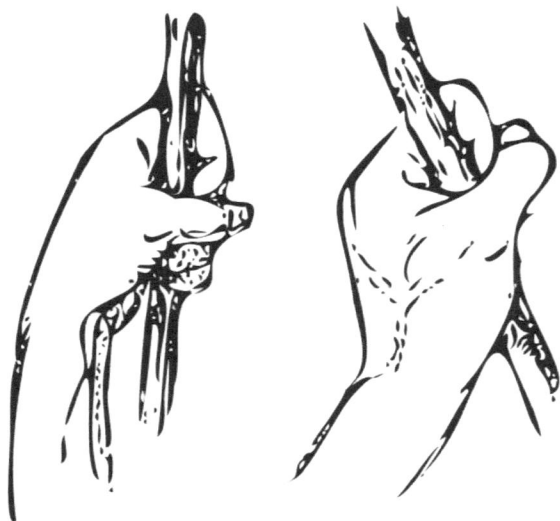

Also the bowhand on the right holds the bow wrongly, for it bends at the wrist. The bowstring would counteract its own launch, the shot going left. Thus the bowhand on the left shows that the wrist must be straight, at most curled a bit outward, as illustrated. (Left is correct and Right is wrong!)

When you upload the arrow—index feather upwards!— hold the bow horizontally, top end rightwards. When the bow is brought upright, the arrow must lay upon the left forefinger. The arrow must form a right angle with the bowstring.

The bow is drawn with forefinger and middle finger, as illustrated. By gripping the arrow between the thumb and forefinger, too many shots launch untimely. Thus you cannot really draw any reasonably heavy bow![28]

Aiming / Readying: The arrow is correctly aimed/ready, when the targeting eye sights it exactly pointing at the target. Thereby shall arrow, left arm, and right elbow align along one plane. The torso must not twist, the back must not crook, and the legs must not wobble.

Drawing / Bending: without bringing arms and arrow out/off level and direction, draw the right hand, bowstring, and arrow to anchor at the chin. Aiming is concerned therewith. Actually, it can even only be improved by the elevation angles. Both eyes are open and see only the target.[29] Tauten all energy, but make nothing convulsive and/or stiff!

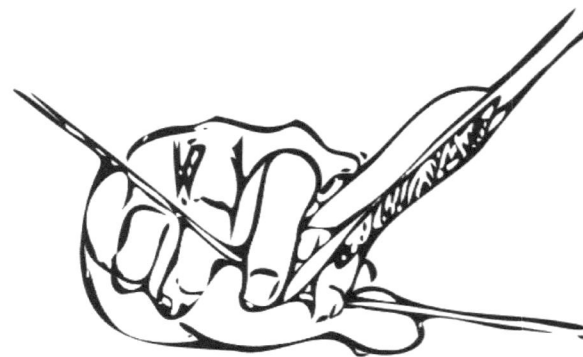

---

[28] You may want to wear something like leather rancher gloves to protect your hands while bowshooting.
[29] This speaks to instinctive archery.

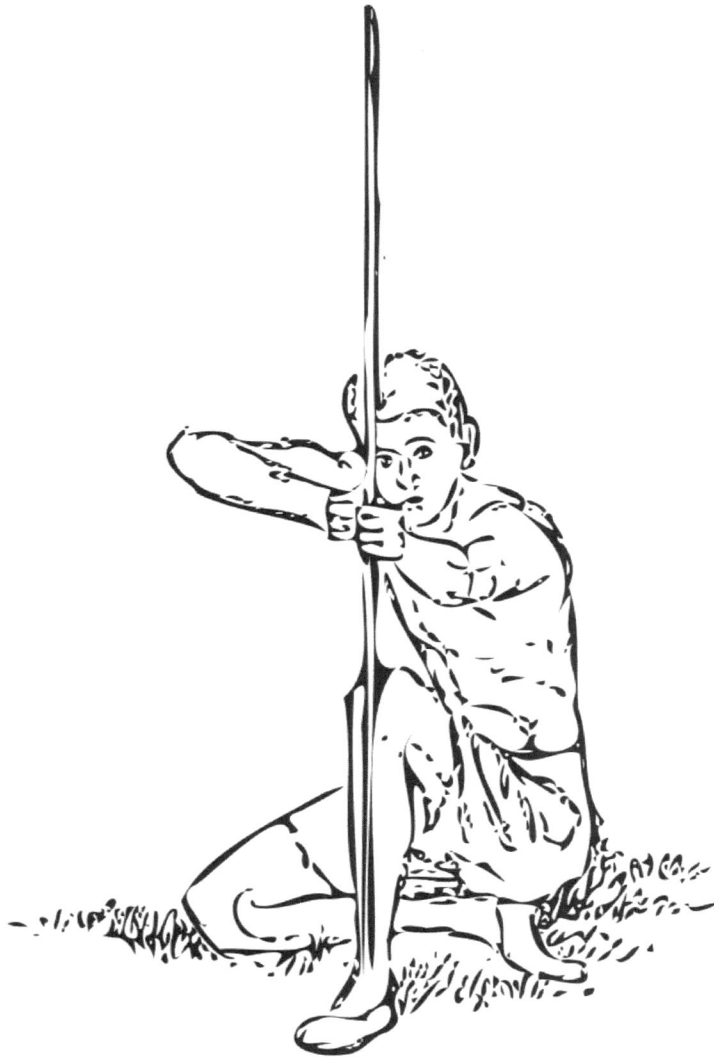

The shot then becomes only just a very quiet movement off the fingertips. Moreover, your whole composure must be maintained ironclad, so that any failed shot can be scrutinized as to what was at fault. As the gunner calmly sights through his muzzle-flash, so the archer calmly checks his arrow and only releases upon command. Short bows let you shoot very well kneeling. The body sways less.

You must simply be very careful that the bottom end of the bow does not strike against the ground due to haste. Then there is breakage!

A variation, which especially makes for fun and yet requires some artistry, is shooting from the back of a comrade e.g. thus across a hedge, or even just for practice. But that is only something for tough and nimble physiques. Other physiques jeopardize the weapon (and both shooter and bearer), and definitely hit nothing.

When shooting upwards—e.g. at advertising balloons, which initially you had better get somewhat used—the arrow must be prevented from slipping off sidewards by the outstretched forefinger of the left hand, as illustrated here.

Prone shooting is very hard! For right-handed shooters the upper bowhorn points leftwards, so that the horizontal-lying bow is seized with an undergrip. The correct elevation is not entirely easy to gain with propped-up elbows. The arrow glides slightly sideways off course.

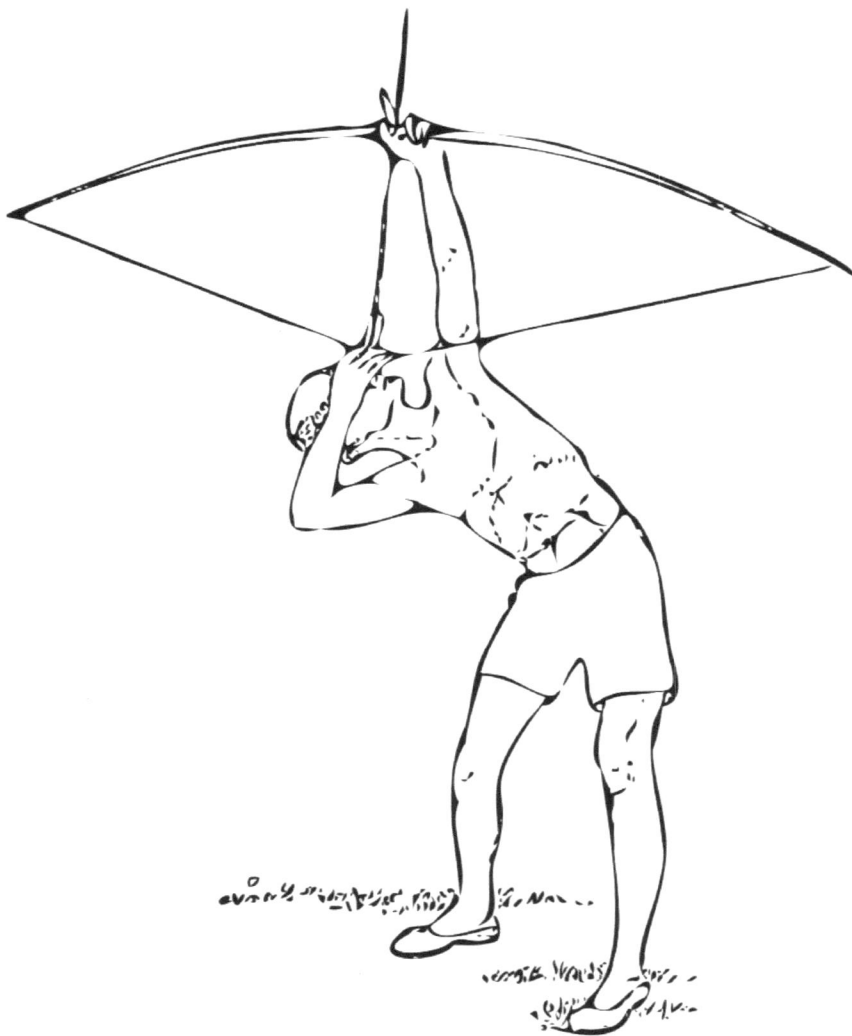

You must totally lay upon your left side so you can aim and draw, as illustrated. Anyway, bowshooting while prone is jolly good training for tenacity and skill; and is needed preparatory training for shooting out from a tree; although the crown of the art of archery, which at least for us we have scant occasion, is to plant our arrows behind the bladebone of a raging buffalo from the saddle of a galloping horse.[30]

Shooting Lessons

At the beginning of all bowshooting, you always provide the youth the needed weapon knowledge, whereby they handle/treat the bow correctly, and know its strengths and weaknesses. Then precisely as normal come the proper gripping and aiming. Naturally and initially, you seek out windless days.

The question of the correct elevation, so to reach the target via your own spanning ability, is difficult enough even without wind.

---

[30] WF probably refers to hunting by American Indian horse-archers across the Great Plains; or perhaps even by Hunnish horse-archers across the Eurasian Steppes.

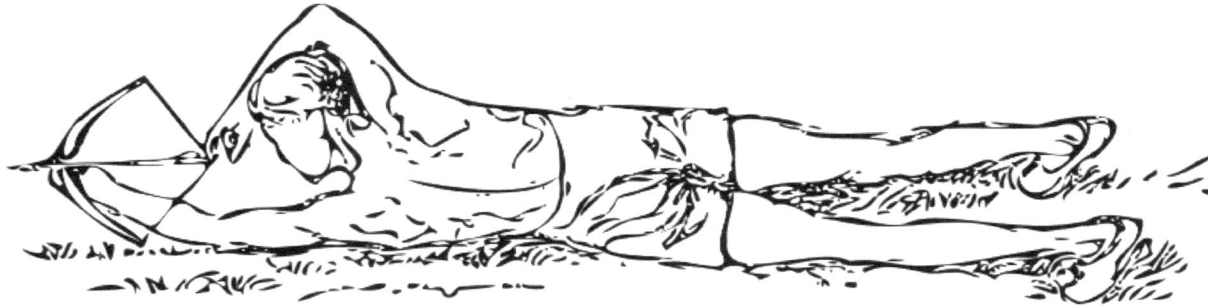

(Whoever can draw the bow up to the "joint"—which is the base of the point of the arrow—he can shoot flat-trajectory across the practice-range. Whoever can only draw to half-arrow length, must naturally make higher/steeper shots.) During wind, flat-trajectory shooting must surely go. The longer the distance, the lighter the weight, and the slower the flight-speed of the arrow; then the greater the wind-effect. Thus during windy weather, try for shorter distances with heavy arrows and flat-trajectory shots. During strong headwinds, do not tilt the target too steeply—because the arrows come down almost vertically from above!

After all the arrows are shot—then fetch every one of the arrows! However, when arrow-fetching is combined with footracing; then the shafts naturally get partly trodden underfoot, get partly disjointed by ripping out of the target, or come to damage by scuffling. (So do not combine those!)

Safeguards (see Shooting Rules)

Shooting Rules for Archery

1. As with any proficient shooting, tranquility[31] must reign. Every movement of archery requires dominance and uniformity. The fragility of this gear and the danger of this weapon equally-little tolerate any haste, excitement, or disorder.

---

[31] The *Ruhe* advocated for German *Bogenschießen* is functionally identical to the *Zen* advocated for Japanese *Kyūdō!*

2. Each squad, which keeps a bow, must also have a "bowyer" subordinate to Battalion E. The bowyer is responsible for the weapon and its shooting activity. It may only be shot in his presence. Outside the shooting range and regulated shooting, the bow may only be tillered/spanned for repair purposes.

3. Before any shooting: the bows, strings, and spare strings are to be meticulously examined, and small flaws mended forthwith. A good backstop for the targets is to be built. Furthermore, the shooting range must be staked out, and thusly be watched by sentinels, so that no one can interlope unauthorized.

4. The bowyer appoints the arrow-fetcher, who is responsible for carefully loosening the missiles out of target or backstop or ground: So give him time to do that!

5. The bowyer strings the bow and gives it to the first shooter. Every shooter has his own arrows or has gotten them at the beginning of shooting. He himself is responsible for their cleanliness.

6. As soon as a shooter has the bow, he becomes silent. Any distraction leads to misses. Each shooter makes the same shot-series as the other. The bowyer advises and improves. Before the next shooter arrives, it is checked whether the string-middle is still 1/10 of its length away from the bow-arch. Failing this, the string gets newly wound.

7. All spectators, whether or not they belong to the shooters, must halt strictly behind the shooter who is shooting; and also they must not veer forward to the sides; and they must remain outside the range of shots (including range of failed shots) staked out by the bowyer.

8. The sentinels appointed for keeping clear the fairway of the outer shooting range are simultaneously arrow-watchers, who lighten the arrow-fetcher's work, especially in the case of runaway arrows.

9. Shooting at flying targets—paper kites, advertising balloons—must never be shot very steeply upwards and always only with the wind-direction. Vertical arrows coming from above are very hard to see in time! If needed, build a bunker for the target-launcher.

10. Never give any of your squad's bows into the hands of any adult who does not belong to the HY![32]

Now go and learn the archery art like Egil son of Wade, the Zealander, who shot the apple from atop his son's head before the Njaren bailiff, 1000 years before William Tell.

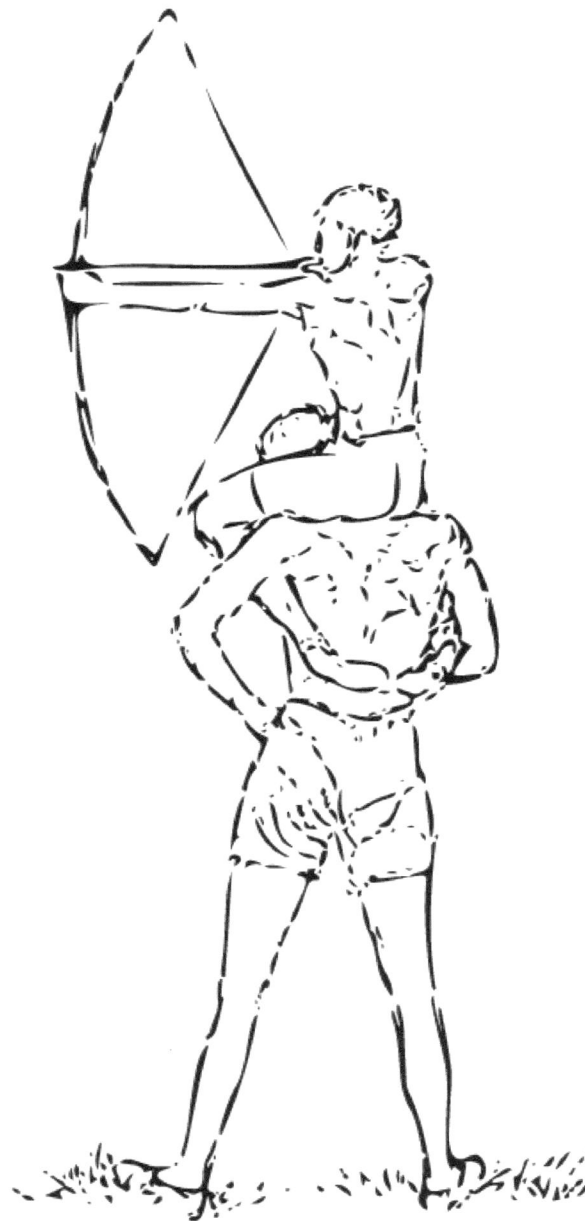

---

[32] This is sound rational advice for any youth, to trust and to deal with only men of his own kind, to retain the weaponized integrity of himself and his fellows. It is safe to presume WF would want this advice extended not only to out-group adults but also to out-group kids; and to retainment of your fencing weaponry as well. Despite the self-destructive advice foisted upon you by degenerate globalists, your instinctive valuing of group and personal sovereignty is both normal and healthy.

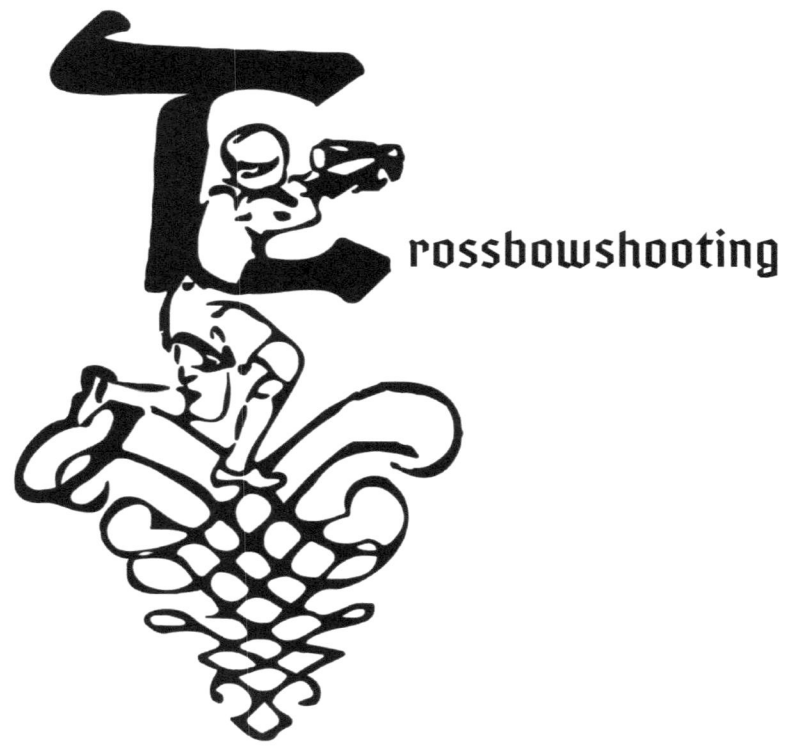

Crossbowshooting

With crossbows, which the Youngfolk can indeed dominate, we have made long shots of 200 meters and have indeed achieved a very decent hit-scores at 100 meters. So our crossbow performs at least as well as a good air-rifle. As a weapon, however, it is for us preferably superior to the air-rifle, since it has not only more punching power, but namely its special character! The shooter sees and senses nothing of the stored and effective pressure of the air-rifle. The propulsion of the crossbow, however, he heavily senses by spanning and by launching, and he sees that too! Plus channeling and mastering a manifested force creates more joy than when some machinery does all the work for you. That is why horseriding is finer than sportscar-driving; and crossbowshooting is finer than blunderbuss-blasting.

The Youngfolk Crossbow 1935

The Bow

Let us get a portion, or better several, of bandsaw-steel from a mechanic, some 60-70 cm long. Old leaf-springs from car or wagon also work, broken but lighter. Smith/Forge the horns, as illustrated by (C1), thusly, so that the bowstring loops tight and smooth. Wagon leaf-springs usually have a square hole in the middle. Through this an eye-screw (A) must pass, which gets affixed to the front of the barrel, whereby the bow's apex wraps exactly over the fittingly curved face of the barrel. For other unpierced steel bows, those must indeed go without that.

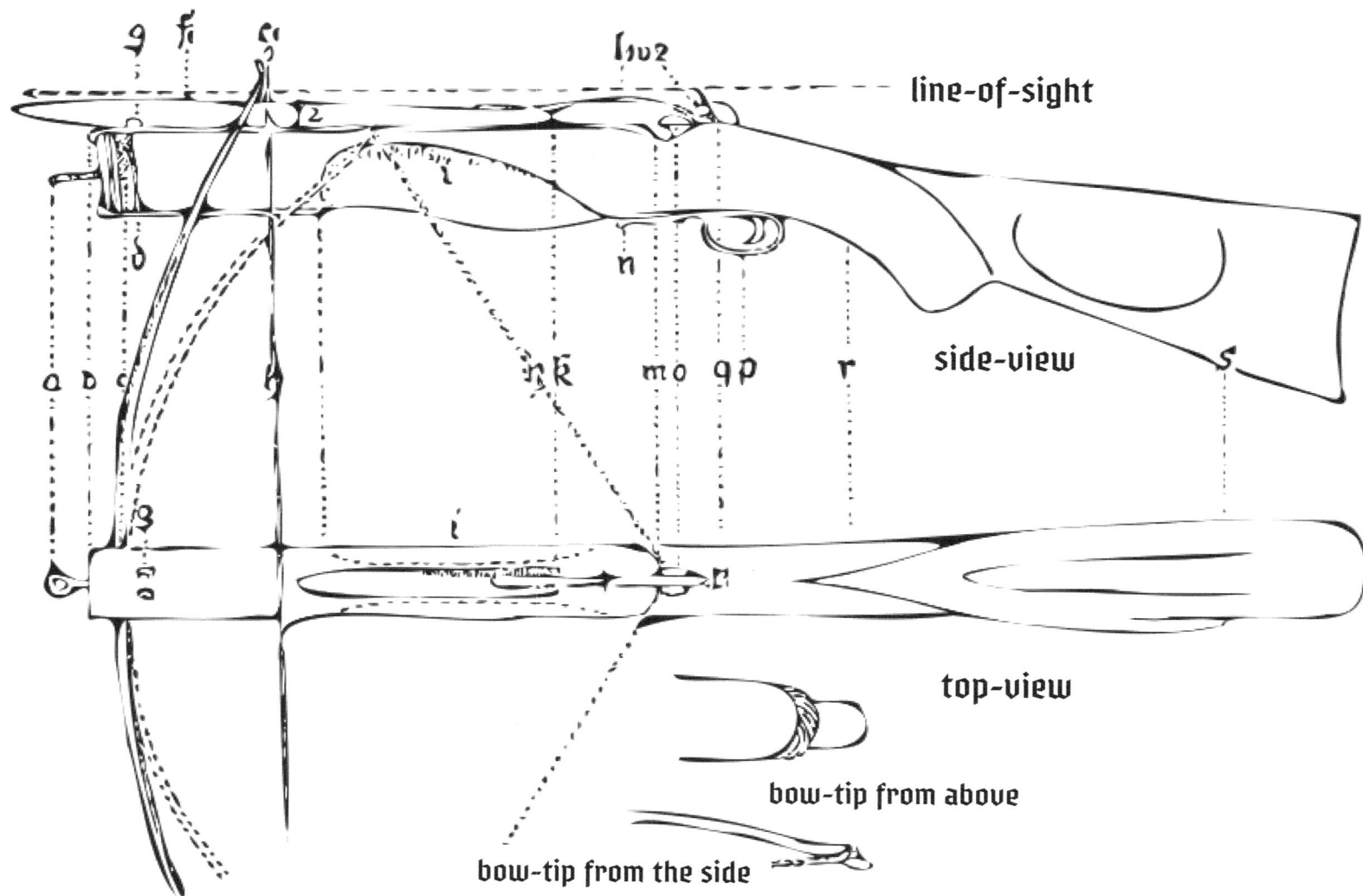

line-of-sight

side-view

top-view

bow-tip from above

bow-tip from the side

Translator's Note: The part-letters range from A to S; for whatever reason, nothing was marked either E or J here, nor T later, and some letters were used twice.

It must then be precisely measured. Via the long and strong eye-screw (A), the faceplate (B) is compressed against the bow, with a leather spacer against the barrel. Without the leather layer, the bow would presumably soon jump because of hard bruising of the wood. The bow must extend slightly slanted, so that the bowstring does not drag too much against the runway and thereby gets braked. The bow shall be rather hard. Soft bows warp and have a great span-width. Thereby the barrel becomes longer, which is awkward for its frontal weight, and you must also carve longer bolts/quarrels.

The String

Gently clamp down the bow-ends to the workbench, so that the bow is slightly taut; then the string is looped over those. It is best to utilize tarred shoemaker-cord or very good waxed twine; and loop this enough times, yet not too tightly, over the bow-horns so that the string becomes 10 mm thick. Then it gets completely wrapped, stroke next to stroke, and additionally well-waxed. Naturally, at the points of contact on the horns, loops are wrapped which you had best heap around twice. But that only works when you do not make the longitudinal winding too tight. Once unclamped and free, the bow must span the string taut, but not too drastically. The bow is now strung and gets no more slackening.

The Barrel

The barrel-length from (D) to (M) concords with the span-width of the bow. So first we must build the spanning lever, as it is illustrated. Then firmly clamp it to the bow in the middle somewhere and make spanning tries. The average width of the attained spannings is the barrel-length between (D) and (M).

You must never let the bow snap back.[33] Thereby the string rips and the bow breaks. The spanning lever needs no further description; only that it must fasten so widely that the barrel is not scarred; and the notches, with which it grabs the string, must be deep and smooth. The illustration shows the barrel-form, which naturally can also be simplified. Firstly, make the stock rather long and then saw it off until it seats comfortably to your frame. The best materials are: walnut, oak, hornbeam, pine/fir, cherry, birch, alder. The barrel has upper and lower fixtures, thus the skids of the crossbow, which are curved a bit in front (claws), so as to hold those fast.

The top skid has a center-trough, the bolt-groove, into which the bolt comes to lay slightly slanted, at its rear end about 3 mm deep. Near the runway-front, a small yoke/clevis is affixed, whereupon the bolt rests just before the center-of-gravity. The bottom skid also has one of the aforesaid claws, and holds bow and faceplate from below. Additionally, some of the lock-parts are set into this bottom skid. You can also even form out the trigger-guard in one piece. However, since the front claws have to hold back the pressure of the bow's anchoring eye-screw (A); then the fixtures must not be weak. It is practical to carve the hand-guard (I) into the barrel, so that the fingers of the left hand do not get over the runway, and then naturally become badly battered.

Spanning Lever

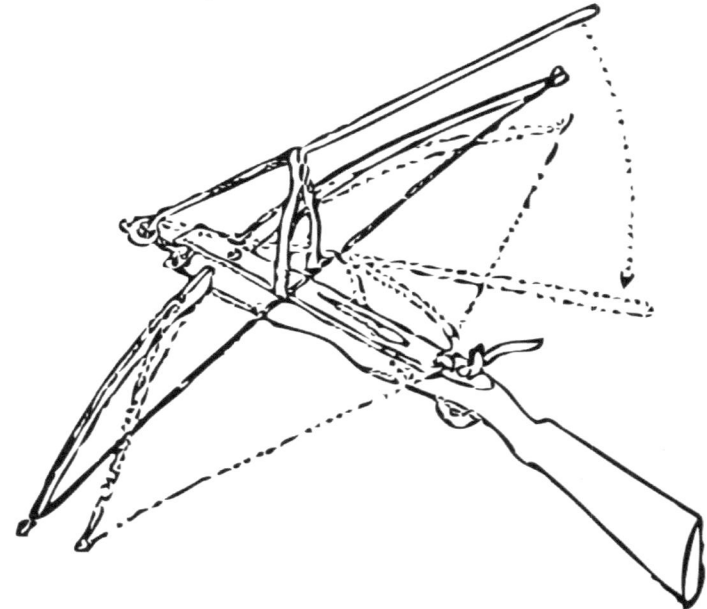

[33] This goes for every crossbow and bow: that you never draw and release any bow which is not loaded with its suitable missile and aimed at a warranted target.

The Bolt

The bolt must have a strength which is reckoned from the thickness of the string and from double the depth of the bolt-groove. It must be hit midway by the quickening string.

It should be front-heavy and rear-light, with center-of-gravity about the front-third. Simple materials: Spruce wood with heavy ferrules. Better and more durable is ash wood. The loaded bolt is held in its position upon the spanned weapon by the clip (L), which gets swiveled sidewards for spanning. This must only lightly rest upon the bolt, because otherwise it crimps during the launch. What is said in archery about the shaft, is accordingly valid for the bolt. Except this missile gets either zero or only two feathers, which affix exactly opposite each other. Also, the bolt does not get any nock; or at most, a shallow filing-out exactly aligned with the two feathers. The more carefully the bolts are crafted, the better are the shooting scores. The bolt must not be too light, because when the load is too low, the string rips and the bow jumps. The bolt-weight depends on the capability of the whole weapon, and so that must be tested. But all bolts should be equally heavy, otherwise a test-series must be shot for each bolt, until their aiming points are determined. If needed, the bolts are numbered, with the aiming point for each number recorded on a ledger.

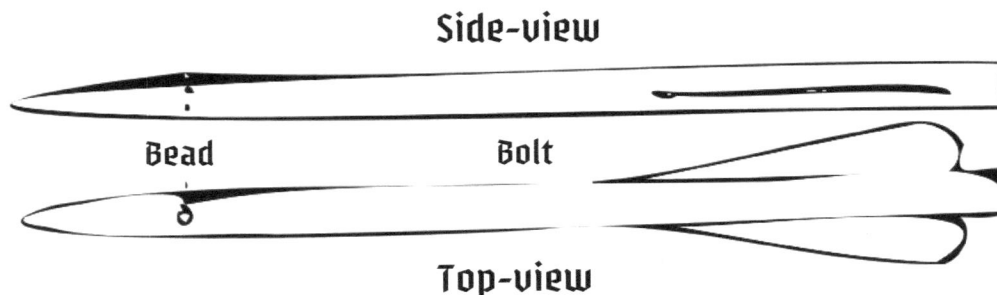

Side-view

Bead   Bolt

Top-view

The Lock

The spanned bowstring goes to sit in the "maw" (M), while it is held fast by the clamp (O). If the clamp is released, the string must be able to glide out easily and without jumping from the "maw."

The Lock

bolt   holding clip   maw

sight
(notch)

safety

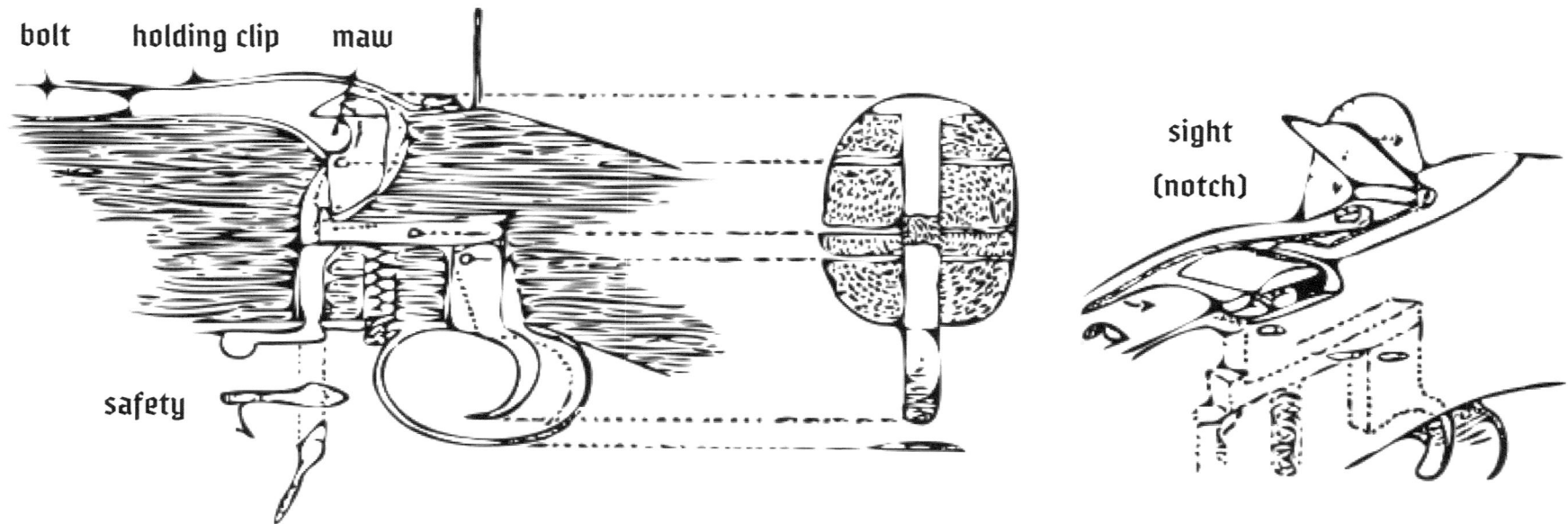

Anyhow, the maw must be just so deep that the pressure of the spanned bowstring on the clamp (O) does not become too great. The clamp itself is held fast in its position by the front claw of the toggle (T). [34] This has a wide top plate, with which it is pressed forward over the string when spanning, until it snaps down into the toggle-claw. The toggle—axle in center—is pressed forward, by a small screw-adjustable spring, against the lower end of clamp (O). Behind lays the toggle upon the top rim of the trigger-body (P2). In this position it can be secured via the cam-roller (N) by flipping this switch under its front-end. Because of the weapon's danger, this safety is strictly needed! It gets opened just immediately before the shot. The launch happens by squeezing back the trigger (P1). Thereby the toggle (T) is lifted at its rear-end and lowered at its front-end. Thus it sets free the bottom end of the clamp (O).

---

[34] Surely all parts are properly illustrated—however, not every mentioned part is fully marked with the proper letters/numbers—thus what was described by WF requires some imagination via his various detailed diagrams.

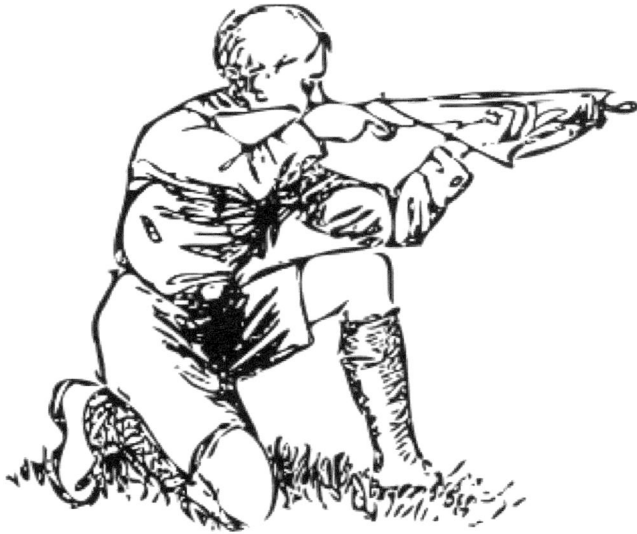

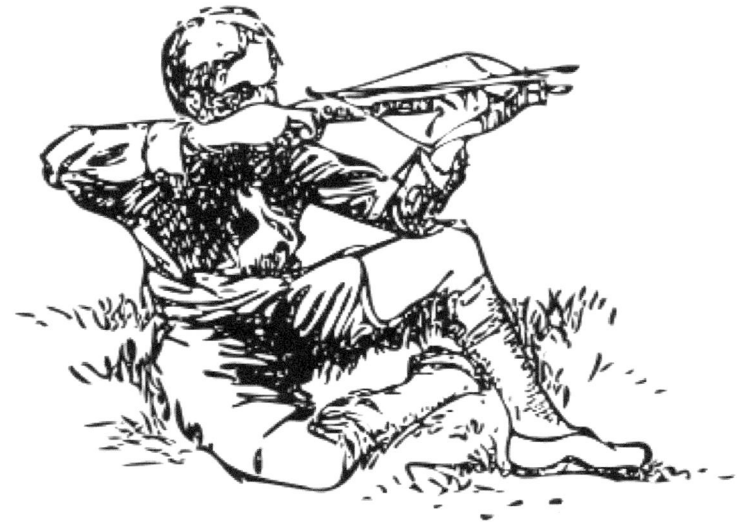

The spanned bowstring squeezes through between the maw-rim and the top skid. We have tested a whole quantity of simplified locks. They all have some disadvantage: Maybe the trigger pulls heavily—then either you accustom to ripping through the string and wrecking your shooting technique—or the string gets too badly frayed, often torn, and usually also shatters the bow. Maybe instead the trigger-track is either too long or too short. In any event, the design illustrated here has the greatest similarity to the ratios for that of the rifle, and spares the string.

The Sighting Mechanism

The bead is a tiny round-headed tack that gets punched into the highest point of the slightly slanted and loaded bolt. The bead-tacks of all the bolts must abide the same height (F1). We have usually fashioned the sight from a hinge, into one flange of which we have filed a notch. The experiential radial scale for the ranges—one for each bolt-weight—is affixed next to it. The line-of-sight is thus: Eye of the Shooter—Notch (Q)—Bead (F1)—Target.

The target is best made of thick lime wood, poplar wood, or spruce wood. Namely, it must be well-anchored. Behind that must be a proper backstop, so that the missiles can neither splinter nor go astray. We shoot at the Eagle according to the old custom.[35]

The Shooting Range

The best is a roofless small-caliber rifle-shooting range—not covered, because the trajectories of the bolts are rather high. If none such stands within your domain, then one must be marked and barricaded accordingly, as with archery. The bowyer is responsible.

Weapons Provisioning

When enough weapons are ordered, our mechanic can undertake the series-production of serviceable crossbows of the type illustrated. Mail/Post to Youth Domain 2/112, Gerlachsheim in Baden. The cost per unit sold shall amount to about 25 Marks/13 Euro. But when you build your own weapon, it is even better. Then you can make many new inventions; from light "bird-rifles" to the heaviest ballistae; like we built them in the deadly trenches, so as to furnish enemy machine-gun-nests with turtle-grenades, before there were any light mortars issued to our infantry.[36]

Shooting with the Crossbow

Here exactly the same rules prevail as for rifle-shooting. But the crossbow has a great frontal weight. For old arbalests, lead inserts were in the stock for equalization.

---

[35] WF refers to traditional target-shooting competitions, still done today, using a brightly painted wooden target shaped like the Reichsadler (Imperial Eagle)—thus NOT shooting or harming of any of those actual noble birds, which any true German would consider to be a sin against Nature.
[36] WF refers to actions by German and Austro-Hungarian military forces during the First World War (1914–1918).

But then the whole weapon becomes too unwieldy for us. Therefore, initially learn to shoot from the bracket, whereby the weapon is laid forth upon a wooden fork stretching to the ground; then kneeling/sitting; then standing just freehanded. The crossbow must chiefly be "tightened up," like a heavy longrifle. Any tedious aiming is not practical. The bowyer must let the shooter shoulder and unshoulder repeatedly. That is why in crossbowshooting, you learn quick targeting and shooting, without pausing long. Furthermore, the weapon provides you a good rifle-position and a correct body-posture, because without those, every shot misses.

Shooting Rules for Crossbowshooting

1. The bowyer is responsible for weapon, target, backstop, shooting range, and barriers. Without him there is no shooting!

2. The bowyer has the spanning lever. He gives into the hands of the shooter the spanned and secured weapon, or lets him span and secure it. The bolt must only become loaded, when the bowyer has authorized the shot.

3. As soon as the bolt lays upon the weapon, all silence themselves and move as little as possible.

4. It must only be shot upon secure shooting ranges and only at solid targets.

5. All spectators have to halt at least three paces behind the shooter or outside the shooting range. That is strictly to prevail!

6. Always only one bolt-gatherer gets dispatched, who carefully loosens the missiles out of targets and so forth, so that they remain usable: So give him time to do that!

GOOD BOLTS!

BIBLIOGRAPHY

Primary Source

Fabricius, Wilhelm. *Ritterliche Waffenspiele, Schwert- und Stockfechten, Bogenschießen, Armbrustschießen, Bau von Übungswaffen etc.*, 2nd Edition. Stuttgart: Holzinger, 1935.

Other Sources

Ahrens, Rüdiger. *Die Bündische Jugend: eine Neue Geschichte 1918-1933.* Göttingen: Wallstein, 2015.

Anonymous. *Master-at-Arms Badge for Boy Scouts.* Glasgow: James Brown and Son, 1926.

Bahro, Berno. *Der Sport und seine Rolle in der Nationalsozialistischen Elitetruppe SS,* Vol.32:1. Historical Social Research; 2007.

Betts, James. *The Sword and How to Use It.* London and Aldershot: Gale and Polden, 1908.

Björn Rüther. "Physics of the Wrath—the Zornhau." YouTube. August 2017.

Bulanda, Edmund. *Bogen und Pfeil bei den Völkern des Altertums.* Wien and Leipzig: Alfred Hölder, 1913.

Coesfeld, Marcus. *Kampfsport im Dritten Reich—Ideologische Instrumentalisierung.* Ruhr-Universität Bochum, 2011.

Degrelle, Leon. *The Eastern Front: Memoirs of a Waffen SS Volunteer, 1941-1945,* Revised Edition. Newport Beach: Institute for Historical Review, 2014.

Dürer, Albrecht. *Handschrift 26-232.* Nürnberg: Albertina Graphische Sammlung Wien, 1512.

Felső-Eöry, Zoltán Cseresnyés. *Safe Outcome of the Sabre-Duel*(1901), Revised Edition, Translated by Krisztina Nagy, Edited by Jeffrey Hull. Academia.edu, 2015.

Gassmann, Jack, Jürg Gassmann and Dominique Le Coultre. *Fighting with the Longsword: Modern-Day HEMA Practices.* Acta Periodica Duellatorum, 2017.

Von Görne, 1st Lt., 2nd Lt. Von Scherff and 2nd Lt. Mertens. *Die Gymnastik und die Fechtkunst in der Armee.* Berlin: A Bath, 1858.

Guts-Muths, Johann. *Turnbuch für die Söhne des Vaterlandes.* Frankfurt am Main: Gebrüdern Wilmans, 1817.

Hull, Jeffrey. *Early European Longswords: Evidence of Form and Function.* Ragnarok Works, 2012.

Hull, Jeffrey. *Inthereof: the Tactical Key to German Fencing,* 4th Edition. Ragnarok Works, 2016.

Hull, Jeffrey. *Mass in Medieval German Fighting Arts,* 3rd Edition. Ragnarok Works, 2016.

Hunt, W Ben. *The Golden Book of Indian Crafts and Lore,* 1st Edition. New York: Golden Press, 1954.

Jahn, Friedrich, Ernest Wilhelm and Bernhard Eiselen. *Die Deutsche Turnkunst zur Einrichtung der Turnplätze dargestellt.* 1816.

Jung, Carl Gustav. "Essay on Wotan." in *Essays on Contemporary Events,* Translated by Barbara Hannah. London: 1947.

Jünger, Ernst. *Storm of Steel (In Stahlgewittern)* (1920), Translated by Michael Hofmann, Foreword by Karl Marlantes. New York: Penguin Classics, 2016.

Klee, Gotthold. *Rittergeschichten für das Deutsche Volk und die Reifere Jugend.* Gütersloh: Bertelsmann, 1906.

Maes, Fritz. *Chivalric Arts of Germany.* Bayern and Oregon: Ragnarok Works, 2016.

Meyer, Joachim. *Gründtliche Beschreibung der Freyen Ritterlichen unnd Adelichen Kunst des Fechtens.* Straßburg: 1570 and 1600.

Oakeshott, Ewart. *Records of the Medieval Sword,* Revised Editon. Woodbridge: Boydell Press, 2002.

Odin. "Deutsche Jungens auf Fahrt '34." YouTube. June 2017.

Odin. "Jungenschaft im Hochlandlager Windham, New York '37." YouTube, June 2017.

Ravenstein, August. *Volksturnbuch: im Sinne von Jahn, Eiselen und Spieß und nach den in Berlin etc.* Frankfurt: Sauerländer, 1876.

Rosenberg, Alfred. *The Myth of the 20th Century (Mythus des XX. Jahrhunderts): an Evaluation of the Spiritual-Intellectual Confrontations of Our Age* (1937), Translated by Peter Peel. Wentzville MO: Invictus Books, 2011.

Rüther, Martin. *Jugend! Deutschland 1918-1945.* NS-Dokumentationszentrums der Stadt Köln. NRW-Landeszentrale für politische Bildung. Landschaftsverband Rheinland: Thyssen Stiftung, 2017.

Sandkühler, Margarete. *Wilhelm Fabricius / Fabricius.* Biographien Dokumentation. Vorschungsstelle Kulturimpuls, 2010.

Simon, Hans. *Der Deutschen Jugend Sportbuch.* Leipzig and Berlin: BG Teubner, 1913.

Stewart's Fencing Coaching Stuff. "Setting Up a Counter Parry or Stop Cut." YouTube, May 2014.

Survival Lilly. "My Bow And Arrow Technique." YouTube, December 2015.

Talhoffer, Hans. *Fechtbuch,* Cod. icon 394a. Bayerische Staatsbibliothek München, 1467.

Theodiskfolk. "Children of the Sun." YouTube. October 2016.

Theodiskfolk. "Deutsche Jugend." YouTube. April 2017.

Theodiskfolk. "Jungbannfahnenweihe." YouTube. March 2017.

Theodiskfolk. "Körperbilder." YouTube. June 2012.

Bibliography of Wilhelm Fabricius (1894-1989)

Wild und Wildlinge. 1927

Führer durch die Gräflich v. Berckheim'schen Anlagen Ausländischer Holzarten in Weinheim a. d. Bergstraße. 1933

Ritterliche Waffenspiele. 1935

Schloßpark und Exotenwald: Weinheim an der Bergstraße; 100 Jahre Fremdländische Baumarten in Weinheim. ca. 1960

Die Rappenreiter. 1970

Der Page und das Paradies. 1976

Geister und Abergeister. 1981

Wunder zwischen Wald und Wasser. 1982

Reiter und Pan. 1982

Die Liebe Gottes. 1985

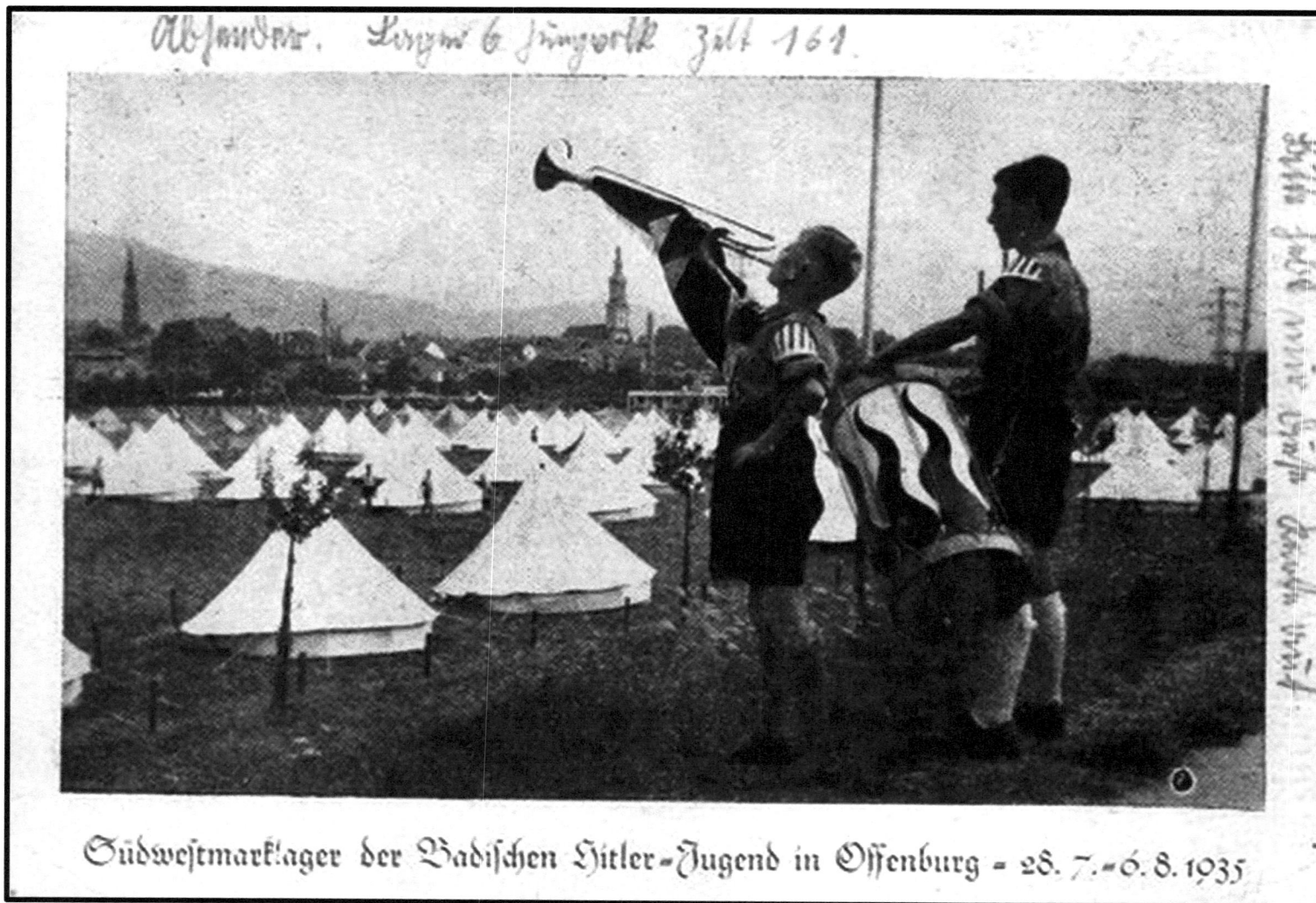

Photograph of the morning call at the Southwestern March Camp (Jamboree) of the Baden Hitler-Youth held near Offenburg during July 28th–August 8th, 1935: This is where and when the fencing and archery of Fabricius enjoyed massive play and proof by Scouts.

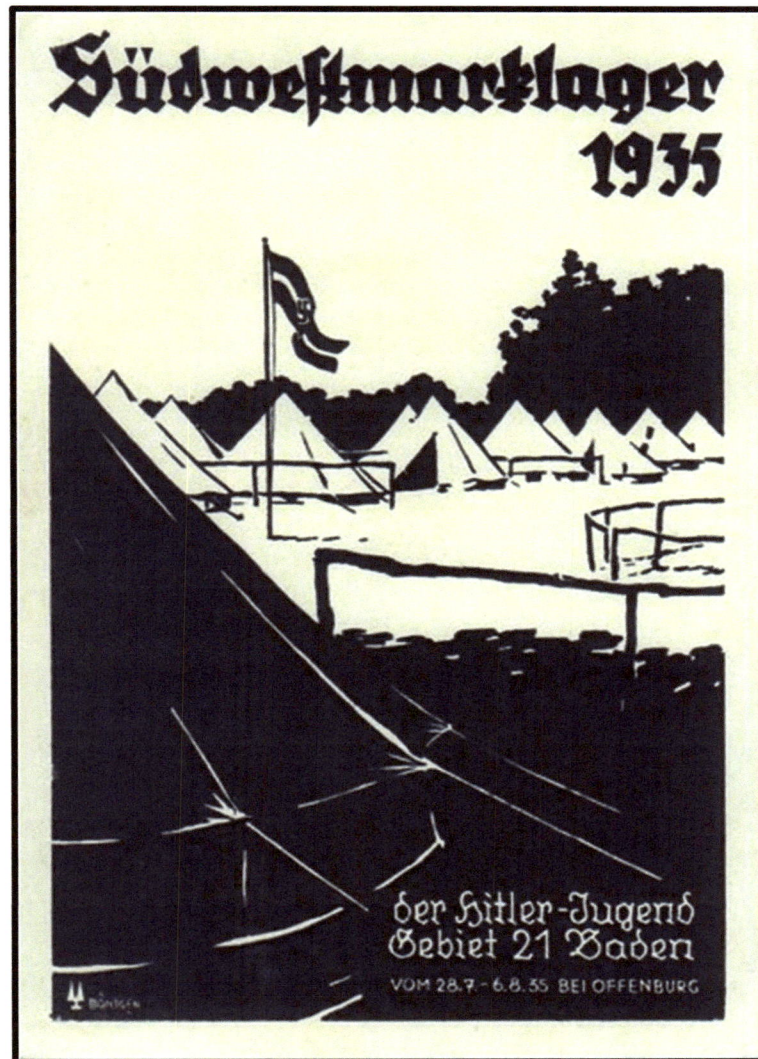

Postcard for the Southwestern March Camp (Jamboree)

www.ingramcontent.com/pod-product-compliance
Lightning Source LLC
Chambersburg PA
CBHW041653260326

41914CB00018B/1625

9781953730954